Emergency

Nursing Care

The Complete Guide

ALEXANDRE CAREWELL

Table of contents

« Emergency isn't just a department, it's the place where medical bravery meets humanity in its purest form, transforming chaos into hope. »

Chapter 1:
INTRODUCTION TO EMERGENCIES

History of the emergency department

Let's take a step back in time, to a time when the concept of emergency medicine had not yet been established. The history of emergency services, like that of medicine, is rich, complex and studded with developments that have shaped our current understanding of fast, effective medical care.

In the early days, there was no emergency department as we know it today. Before the advent of modern medicine, most medical care was provided in the home. Doctors travelled from house to house, treating their patients at the bedside, often in the absence of specialised equipment or advanced knowledge. If a situation required immediate intervention, it was managed on the spot, often with limited resources.

However, with the industrial revolution and increasing urbanisation of the 19th and 20th centuries, hospitals began to play a central role in the provision of care. Machine-related injuries, accidents and sudden ailments required a dedicated place where patients could be treated quickly. And so the first emergency services were born. Initially, these services were rudimentary, but they performed a vital function, becoming the front line of hospital medicine.

Developments in medical techniques and research have also influenced the growth and sophistication of the emergency department. Advances in anaesthesia, surgery and radiology have enabled rapid interventions that were previously unthinkable. Similarly, the advent of ambulances and pre-hospital services has revolutionised patient care, enabling immediate care and safe transport to medical centres.

Over the decades, the emergency department has become increasingly professional. The nurse has become a central figure, combining technical competence, compassion and speed of action. Specialised training for both doctors and nurses has become the norm, and protocols have been developed to deal effectively with a multitude of situations.

Today, emergency departments around the world are bastions of emergency medicine, where every second counts. Millions of lives are saved every year thanks to the rapid, expert and coordinated intervention of medical teams. Looking back, we can appreciate how far we've come and recognise the countless anonymous heroes who have contributed to the evolution of this vital service.

The story of the Emergency Department is not just the story of a medical speciality, but the story of our humanity in the face of the fragility of life. It reminds us of our ongoing commitment to preserving life, fighting disease and offering hope and healing to those who need it most.

The role and importance of emergency departments in the healthcare system

Medical emergencies have always existed, but it is through medical and technological advances that the emergency department has become a central pivot in the healthcare system. Occupying a unique position, it is the gateway for many patients in distress, becoming the first line of defence against illness, injury or deteriorating health.

From the moment a patient walks through the emergency door, a well-oiled machine is set in motion. The service has to respond rapidly to a wide range of pathologies, from minor injuries to life-and-death situations. In this fast-paced environment, the emergency department plays a number of essential roles:

- **Triage and initial assessment:** This is often the first point of contact for the patient. Healthcare professionals assess the seriousness of the situation and determine the priority for treatment.
- **Stabilising patients:** In critical situations, the first objective is to stabilise the patient, whether in respiratory distress, haemorrhage or another life-threatening emergency.
- **Diagnosis and referral:** Thanks to specialised equipment and skills, emergency teams are able to make rapid diagnoses, enabling patients to be referred appropriately, whether for hospitalisation, surgery or other specialised services.
- **Role as guardian of the healthcare system:** In many regions, particularly those lacking access to regular primary care, the emergency department becomes by default the main provider of care for a diverse population. It responds not only to medical emergencies, but also to non-emergency needs for which patients often don't know where to turn.
- **Training and research:** Emergency departments are also training centres for doctors, nurses and other healthcare professionals. In addition, being at the forefront of medical challenges, they play a key role in clinical research, constantly seeking ways to improve emergency care.

The emergency department is therefore much more than just a place for medical care. It is a reflection of society in all its diversity and complexity. It embodies urgency, hope and resilience, playing an indispensable role in the continuum of healthcare.

What's more, its importance extends beyond its walls. Emergency departments influence health policy, hospital budgets and large-scale care planning. Every decision taken, every innovation adopted in this department has repercussions for the rest of the healthcare system.

Emergency departments are a constant reminder that, when faced with the uncertainty and fragility of life, the rapid, competent and caring response of a dedicated team can mean the difference between life and death. This is what makes emergency departments such a vital and revered pillar of the modern healthcare system.

The day-to-day life
of an emergency nurse:
Challenges and rewards

When an ambulance siren sounds or a door suddenly opens to let a stretcher through, the emergency nurse is already in action mode, ready to face the unexpected. This thrilling daily routine is a mixture of adrenaline, skill, empathy and resilience.

Challenges
- **Diversity of cases:** Unlike other specialities, emergency nurses must be prepared to deal with an impressive range of pathologies - from fractures to heart attacks, unexpected deliveries to serious infections. This diversity requires constant adaptability and regular updating of skills.
- **Steady pace:** Days can be unpredictable. There may be moments of calm followed by hours of intense chaos, where every second counts.

- **Emotional management:** In the face of pain, distress or even death, nurses must demonstrate great emotional strength. They are often the first point of contact for patients and their families, offering comfort and reassurance even in the darkest moments.
- **Interprofessional collaboration:** Emergency departments are places where coordination with other health professionals - doctors, radiologists, surgeons, etc. - is essential. - is essential. This collaboration must be fluid, even in times of stress.
- **Physical demands:** Standing for long hours, moving quickly and handling patients all require good physical condition. Exposure to infectious diseases can also be a risk.

Awards
- **Immediate impact:** Emergency nurses often see the direct results of their intervention, whether it's stabilised breathing, relieved pain or a life saved.
- **Constant learning:** The variety of cases offers an unrivalled learning opportunity, making every day a chance to acquire new skills or knowledge.
- **A deep bond with patients:** Although contact may be brief, the intensity of the situations often creates deep and meaningful bonds with patients and their families.
- **Team spirit:** Working in such a dynamic environment forges strong bonds with colleagues. Camaraderie and mutual support are often the keys to overcoming the toughest challenges.
- **Job satisfaction:** Despite the challenges, many nurses talk about the deep sense of fulfilment they get from knowing that they make a real difference to people's lives every day.

The role of the emergency nurse is far from easy, yet it is one of the most rewarding in the medical field. By skilfully balancing challenges and rewards, these healthcare professionals embody the very spirit of dedication, competence and humanity, making them invaluable pillars in the world of medicine.

Chapter 2:
THE EMERGENCY ENVIRONMENT

The sorting room: The first stage

• Severity criteria

In the hustle and bustle of emergency departments, triage, or the act of prioritising patients according to the seriousness of their condition, is a crucial step. This ensures that patients who present the most serious risks are cared for first. To do this, triage nurses use precisely defined severity criteria. These criteria vary according to the symptoms presented, but several of them are universally recognised as indicators of a potentially dangerous situation.

- **Abnormal vital signs:** Values outside the norm for blood pressure, heart rate, respiratory rate, temperature or oxygen saturation may indicate a serious condition.
- **Respiratory distress:** Shallow, wheezy, rapid or laboured breathing is always a cause for concern. The inability to speak in complete sentences may also be an indicator.
- **Chest pain:** Chest pain, especially if accompanied by other symptoms such as sweating, nausea or shortness of breath, may suggest a heart attack or other serious heart problem.
- **Altered mental state:** Sudden confusion, disorientation, dizziness, fainting or changes in level of consciousness are worrying signs.
- **Neurological signs:** Symptoms such as sudden weakness on one side of the body, slurred speech,

blurred vision or severe headaches may indicate a stroke or other serious neurological condition.
- **Heavy bleeding:** Whether internal or external, uncontrolled bleeding can quickly become life-threatening.
- **Severe abdominal pain:** Intense or persistent pain may be a sign of conditions such as appendicitis, bowel obstruction or organ rupture.
- **Severe allergic reactions:** The rapid onset of symptoms such as itching, swelling, breathing difficulties or shock following exposure to an allergen is a medical emergency.
- **Signs of severe infection:** High fever associated with chills, tachycardia, hypotension or lethargy may indicate sepsis or another serious infection.
- **Trauma:** Injuries resulting from accidents, falls or violence, depending on their location and severity, may require immediate treatment.

These criteria are just the tip of the iceberg. In reality, the ability to assess severity is also based on clinical experience, professional intuition and ongoing training. The assessment skills of an experienced emergency nurse are a blend of science and art, and play an invaluable role in saving lives.

• Communication with waiting patients
Emergency departments, with their hectic pace and busy atmosphere, can be a source of anxiety for many patients. Waiting is often the worst time for them, filled with uncertainty, discomfort and stress. In this context, communication becomes an invaluable tool for calming, informing and managing expectations. Here's how it works for an emergency nurse.

- **Establishing trust from the outset:** During the first interaction, the nurse must establish a climate of trust. This involves active listening, eye contact and reassuring gestures. Introducing yourself and briefly explaining your role can also help to build trust.
- **Explain the triage process:** Many patients do not understand why others who arrive after them are seen first. Explaining the concept of triage based on case severity can help clarify the situation and minimise frustration.
- **Regular updates:** If a patient has a long wait, it's essential to keep them informed of the situation. A simple "We haven't forgotten, but we're overloaded at the moment" can alleviate some concerns.
- **Be clear and honest:** If tests or procedures are to be carried out, it is crucial to explain what they are, why they are necessary and how long they will take.
- **Actively listening to concerns:** Some patients have specific needs or concerns during the wait. These may relate to pain, anxiety or personal problems such as childcare. By listening, you can find solutions or offer support.
- **Use appropriate   language:** While maintaining medical precision, it is essential to express yourself in a way that is simple and understandable to the patient. Avoid medical jargon wherever possible and make sure that the patient has understood the information.
- **Managing emotions:** Some patients can become agitated, anxious or even angry. It is essential to approach these situations with empathy, calm and professionalism, while setting clear limits.
- **Reassurance about care:** Even while waiting, patients need to know that they are in good hands and that their well-being is a priority.
- **Encourage feedback:** Asking patients how to improve communication or the waiting process can

provide valuable information for optimising the service.

Effective, empathetic communication not only reduces patient anxiety, it also promotes better cooperation, minimises misunderstandings and builds trust in healthcare professionals. In the world of emergency departments, where every moment can be crucial, good communication with waiting patients is an invaluable asset in ensuring that care is provided smoothly and efficiently.

The treatment room

• Basic medical equipment

The medical world of the emergency department is a mixture of rapid action, precise diagnosis and technical procedures. To carry out these tasks, nurses rely on a wide range of medical equipment. These tools, essential to patient care, must be both reliable and rapidly accessible. Here is an overview of the basic medical equipment typically found in an emergency department.

- **Vital signs monitor:** This device is used to monitor the patient's blood pressure, heart rate, respiratory rate, temperature and oxygen saturation, either continuously or on an ad hoc basis.
- **The defibrillator:** Vital for treating cardiac arrest, it sends an electrical impulse to the heart in an attempt to restore a normal heart rhythm.
- **The emergency trolley (or resuscitation trolley):** This contains all the equipment needed for cardiopulmonary resuscitation, such as medicines, syringes, endotracheal tubes and many other essential tools.

- **Mucus aspirator:** Used to remove secretions from the mouth or respiratory tract, it is essential during operations to clear the airways.
- **Pulse oximeter:** Usually placed on the fingertip, it measures oxygen saturation in the blood, giving a rapid indication of the patient's lung function.
- **Stethoscope: An** emblematic tool of the medical world, it is used to listen to the internal sounds of the body, such as heartbeats, breathing noises or intestinal sounds.
- **Blood pressure monitor :** Used to measure blood pressure, this tool is essential for assessing a patient's haemodynamic condition.
- **Clinical thermometer:** This comes in different models (ear, forehead and oral) and is crucial for detecting febrile or hypothermic states.
- **Intubation kit:** Used to keep the airway open, it includes laryngoscope blades, endotracheal tubes and cuffs.
- **Syringes and needles:** These come in different sizes and are used to administer medicines and vaccines or to take blood samples.
- **Infusion sets:** These include all the equipment needed to administer intravenous solutions or medicines.
- **Infusion pump:** Used to administer medicines or fluids at a precise rate.
- **Suture material:** Used to suture wounds, it includes needles, threads and forceps.
- **Dressing materials:** Includes compresses, bandages, antiseptics and other essentials to protect and treat wounds.
- **Immobilisation equipment:** Like splints or cervical collars, these are used to immobilise limbs or the spinal column in the event of a suspected fracture or injury.

This equipment, often strategically placed for optimum use, is the basis of emergency care. Nurses must have perfect command of this equipment if they are to be able to intervene quickly and effectively, often in situations where every second counts.

• Room and bed management

The fluidity of the emergency department depends largely on the optimal management of spatial resources. Wards and beds, in particular, are at the heart of this dynamic, as they represent the place where patients receive direct care. Poor management can lead to delays, frustration and even risks to patient safety. Let's take a look at this often underestimated but essential aspect of emergency care.

- **The importance of an effective triage system:** Even before considering ward and bed management, it is essential to triage patients correctly as soon as they arrive. An effective triage system ensures that beds and wards are allocated according to medical priority, not order of arrival.
- **Bed rotation:** Rapid and thorough cleaning and disinfection of beds between patients is essential to prevent the spread of infections. This requires close coordination between the care team and the cleaning team.
- **Capacity management:** In situations where there is a massive influx of patients, such as during disasters or epidemics, emergency departments can quickly become overwhelmed. Having a plan to increase bed capacity, even temporarily, can be vital. This could include using non-traditional areas for care or transferring patients to other wards or hospitals.
- **Management of specialist beds:** Some beds and wards are specifically equipped for particular types of care, such as trauma or cardiology. The

22

correct allocation of these resources is vital to ensure that patients receive the right care.

- **Interdepartmental communication:** Emergency departments are not isolated. Working closely with other departments, such as radiology, surgery or intensive care, can make it easier to move patients around the hospital.
- **Waiting time management :** Although every effort is made to minimise waiting times, sometimes patients have to wait for a bed. In these situations, clear and empathetic communication is essential to manage expectations and reassure patients.
- **Real-time monitoring technologies:** Many modern hospitals use real-time monitoring systems to visualise bed availability, facilitating decision-making and coordination.
- **Protocols for patients on long waits:** In situations where patients have to wait for long periods for a bed in a specialist unit, clear protocols are needed to ensure that they receive adequate care while waiting.
- **Staff training and education:** Staff should receive regular training on best practice in bed and ward management, as well as specific hospital protocols.
- **Feedback and continuous improvement:** Feedback from healthcare professionals, patients and their families is essential to identify areas for improvement and adapt management strategies.

The efficient management of emergency rooms and beds is a logistical ballet requiring exceptional coordination, communication and preparation. When well managed, it enables optimal patient flow, efficient use of resources and fast, effective care, ensuring the best outcome for every patient.

Chapter 3:
ESSENTIAL CLINICAL SKILLS

Rapid patient assessment

• ABCDE of assessment

The ABCDE approach is a systematic triage and assessment tool used by healthcare professionals, particularly in emergency departments, to assess and treat patients in an order that prioritises immediate threats to life. This method ensures that no vital step is omitted in the initial assessment and management of the patient. Let's take a closer look at each of these steps:

- A - Airways
  - **Assessment**: Make sure the airways are clear and that there are no obstructions preventing the flow of air.
  - **Intervention**: If the airway is unsecured or obstructed (by blood, vomit, trauma, etc.), immediate intervention, such as intubation or placing the patient in a safe position, may be necessary.
- B - Breathing
  - **Assessment**: Observe rate and depth of breathing, listen to breath sounds and assess symmetry of chest expansion.
  - **Intervention**: In the event of respiratory distress, the patient may require oxygen therapy, assisted ventilation or other interventions to stabilise breathing.

- C - Traffic
  - **Assessment**: Check pulse, blood pressure, skin colour and temperature. Look for signs of shock or bleeding.
  - **Intervention**: In the event of circulatory problems, interventions such as the administration of fluids, cardiopulmonary resuscitation (CPR) or medication may be required.
- D - Neurological deficit (Disability)
  - **Assessment**: Rapidly assess the neurological state using the Glasgow Scale or other tools to measure the level of consciousness. Check pupil reactivity, motor skills and sensation.
  - **Intervention**: Depending on the results, action may include stabilisation of the spine, administration of medication or other specialised care.
- E - Exposure/Environment
  - **Assessment**: Examine the whole body, removing clothing if necessary to look for hidden injuries, while preserving the patient's dignity and protecting them from hypothermia.
  - **Intervention**: Treat any wounds discovered, cover the patient to maintain a stable body temperature and protect against other environmental stresses.

After completing the ABCDE assessment, it is crucial to reassess the patient regularly, particularly if their condition changes. This methodology serves as the cornerstone of the initial assessment of patients in an emergency environment, ensuring structured and consistent management and reducing the risk of missing life-threatening situations.

• Interpretation of vital signs

Vital signs are objective measures of basic bodily functions and play an essential role in assessing an individual's physiological state. In the emergency context, their rapid and correct interpretation can often guide initial intervention and provide crucial clues about a patient's state of health. Here is a detailed exploration of these signs and their interpretation:

- Body temperature
    - *Normal*: Average around 37°C, but may vary between 36.1°C and 37.2°C.
    - *Interpretation*: A high temperature (fever) may indicate infection, inflammation or other medical conditions. A low body temperature (hypothermia) may result from exposure to cold, certain illnesses or hypothyroidism.
- Pulse or Heart Rate
    - *Normal*: 60-100 beats per minute (bpm) for an adult at rest.
    - *Interpretation*: A high heart rate (tachycardia) may be caused by fever, anaemia, dehydration or other conditions. A low heart rate (bradycardia) may be due to hypothermia, medication or heart problems.
- Respiratory rate
    - *Normal*: 12-20 breaths per minute for an adult at rest.
    - *Interpretation*: Rapid respiratory rate (tachypnoea) may be due to fever, anxiety, anaemia or lung disease. Slow breathing (bradypnoea) may be caused by medication, brain damage or other conditions.
- Blood Pressure
    - *Normal*: Systolic 90-120 mmHg, Diastolic 60-80 mmHg for an adult.
    - *Interpretation*: High blood pressure (hypertension) is a risk factor for many

cardiovascular diseases. Low blood pressure (hypotension) may indicate dehydration, blood loss or other serious medical conditions.

- Oxygen saturation (SpO2)
  - *Normal*: 95-100%.
  - *Interpretation*: An SpO2 of less than 95% may indicate hypoxaemia, which means that oxygen levels in the blood are insufficient. This may be due to lung or heart problems or severe anaemia.
- Pain
  - Although technically not a 'vital sign' in the traditional sense, pain assessment is often included as a fifth vital sign.
  - *Interpretation*: The pain scale, generally ranging from 0 (no pain) to 10 (worst pain imaginable), helps clinicians assess the intensity of a patient's pain, understand the potential cause and decide what interventions are necessary.

When interpreting vital signs, it is essential to take into account the patient's overall context, including age, gender, medical history and other symptoms present. Slight variations may be normal for some individuals, while larger or sudden deviations often require medical attention and intervention.

Intervention techniques

• Placement of venous lines

Inserting a peripheral venous line, commonly known as an "intravenous catheter" or "perfusion line", is a common procedure in the medical field, particularly in emergency departments. It is used to administer medicines and fluids and to take blood samples. Here is a detailed overview of the procedure:

- Preparation
    - **Choice of equipment**: Selection of the catheter according to its intended use (administration of drugs, solutions, samples) and the size of the patient's veins.
    - **Preparing the patient**: Informing the patient of the procedure, reassuring them and obtaining their consent. Position the arm appropriately.
    - **Hygiene**: Wash your hands and wear sterile gloves.
- Selecting the insertion site
    - Common sites include the veins on the back of the hand, the forearm and the crease of the elbow.
    - Selection depends on the size and condition of the veins and the patient's comfort. Avoid sites near joints, if possible, to reduce catheter mobility.
- Disinfection
    - Use a compress soaked   in antiseptic to disinfect the insertion site, using circular movements from the inside outwards.
- Catheter   insertion
    - Tighten the skin to stabilise the vein.
    - Insert the needle following the path of the vein, at the appropriate angle (usually between 10° and 30°).
    - When venous return is observed in the catheter chamber, move forward slightly more, then insert the catheter while withdrawing the needle.
- Mounting and use
    - Fix the catheter   firmly to the skin with adhesive tape or special devices to prevent movement.
    - Place a sterile   compress over the insertion point. Then connect the infusion system or the infusion stopper.

- Start administering medication or fluids as prescribed.
- Maintenance and surveillance
  - Check the insertion site regularly for signs of infection, inflammation, haematoma or infiltration.
  - Make sure that the infusion rate is correct and that the patient shows no signs of discomfort or complications.
- Withdrawal
  - Stop the infusion.
  - Gently withdraw the catheter in the direction of the vein, applying gentle pressure with a compress to prevent bleeding.
  - Observe and assess the insertion site. If everything seems normal, secure the compress with adhesive tape.

Inserting a venous line requires a skilful technique and a careful approach to minimise the risk of complications and ensure patient comfort.

• Intubation and ventilation

Endotracheal intubation is a medical procedure that involves inserting a tube into the trachea to allow mechanical ventilation of the lungs. This procedure can be vital in situations where the patient is unable to maintain an adequate airway or vent on their own. Here is a detailed overview of the procedure and what happens next:

- Indications for intubation
  - Acute respiratory failure.
  - Protection of the airways (for example, in the event of trauma or poisoning).
  - Surgical procedures requiring general anaesthesia.
  - Cardiorespiratory arrest.

- Preparation
  - **Choice of equipment**: Prepare the appropriate size laryngoscope, endoscope and endotracheal tube.
  - **Medication**: Sedation and paralysis agents may be required to facilitate intubation.
  - **Patient position** : Sniffing position, with extension of the neck and flexion of the head.
- Intubation procedure
  - Open the patient's mouth and carefully insert the laryngoscope.
  - Expose the vocal cords by gently elevating the epiglottis with the blade of the laryngoscope.
  - Insert the endotracheal tube through the vocal cords into the trachea.
  - Remove the laryngoscope while holding the tube in place.
- Confirmation of tube position
  - Observe the symmetrical elevation of both hemithoraxes during ventilation.
  - Listen to the breathing sounds on both sides of the chest.
  - Use a capnograph to detect exhaled CO_2, confirming that the tube is in place.
  - A chest X-ray may also be taken to confirm the position.
- Tube fixing and ventilation
  - Attach the tube firmly to the patient's mouth to prevent accidental displacement.
  - Connect the tube to a mechanical ventilator or self-inflating bag for ventilation.
- Post-intubation monitoring
  - Monitor the patient's vital signs, oxygen saturation and tube position regularly.
  - Assess the patient's comfort and sedation and adjust the medication if necessary.

- Extubation
  - Once the underlying causes of intubation have been resolved, the patient can be extubated.
  - Make sure the patient is sufficiently awake, responds to commands, has a good cough reflex and is respiratory stable.
  - Remove the tube quickly while asking the patient to cough to expel any mucus or debris.

Mastery of the intubation technique requires in-depth training and practice, as the procedure presents risks. Particular attention must be paid to preparation, safe performance of intubation and careful monitoring of the intubated patient.

• CPR and defibrillation

Cardiopulmonary resuscitation (CPR) and defibrillation are vital interventions in the event of sudden cardiac arrest. These procedures can considerably increase the patient's chances of survival and recovery without neurological sequelae.

- Recognition of cardiac arrest
  - Lack of response to stimulation.
  - Absence of breathing or abnormal breathing (such as gasps).
  - No pulse.
- Immediate start of CPR
  - **Patient position**: Lay the patient on their back on a hard surface.
  - **Chest compression**: Place your hands on top of each other in the centre of the chest and give deep compressions (at least 5 cm) at a rate of at least 100-120 per minute.
  - **Ventilation**: After 30 compressions, give 2 breaths keeping the airway open, either using

mouth-to-mouth resuscitation or a barrier device.

- Using an automated external defibrillator (AED)
  - Switch on the AED as soon as it is available.
  - Follow the device's voice or visual instructions.
  - Place the electrodes as shown (one under the right collarbone and the other on the lower left side of the chest).
  - Make sure no one is touching the patient while the AED is assessing the heart rhythm.
  - If a shock is recommended, check again that no-one is touching the patient, then press the shock button.
- Continuation of CPR
  - Resume CPR immediately after defibrillation.
  - Alternate chest compressions and ventilation (30:2 ratio).
  - If you are alone, perform CPR for about 2 minutes before checking the rhythm again with the AED.
  - If several rescuers are present, change roles every 2 minutes to avoid fatigue.
- Post-resuscitation
  - If the patient shows signs of returning to spontaneous circulation (such as movement, coughing, taking a breath), stop CPR and assess breathing and pulse.
  - If the patient is breathing normally, put him/her in the lateral safety position.
  - Continuously monitor the patient while waiting for advanced help.
- Advanced care
  - When advanced medical care is available, medication, intubation and other interventions may be required.

- The patient may require intensive care and further investigations to determine the cause of the cardiac arrest.

Rapid response is essential in the event of cardiac arrest. Every minute without CPR and defibrillation significantly reduces the patient's chances of survival. Regular training and simulated emergency scenarios are essential to maintain CPR and defibrillation skills.

Chapter 4:
COMMON PATHOLOGIES AND CARE

Trauma

• Polytrauma

Polytrauma refers to serious injuries that affect several regions or systems of the human body simultaneously. These emergency medical situations require rapid assessment, prioritisation and intervention to optimise the patient's chances of survival and recovery. Here is a detailed overview of the management of polytrauma:

- Initial assessment
    - **ABCDE**: This assessment focuses on airway protection (Airway), breathing (Breathing), circulation (Circulation), neurological deficit (Disability) and exposure/environment (Exposure/Environment).
    - **Stabilisation**: Immediate stabilisation of vital functions is essential before further assessment.
- Secondary assessment
    - **Complete examination**: This phase consists of a head-to-toe examination to identify any injuries.
    - **Imaging**: X-rays, a CT scan or ultrasound may be necessary for a more accurate assessment.
- Airway and breathing   management
    - Intubation may be necessary to protect the airways or ensure adequate ventilation.

- Thoracic trauma, such as pneumothorax or haemopneumothorax, may require thoracostomy or placement of a chest tube.
- Traffic management
  - Controlling external bleeding with compressions, dressings or tourniquets.
  - Internal bleeding may require surgical or radiological intervention for stabilisation.
- Neurological assessment and management
  - Monitoring and stabilisation of neurological function, assessment of level of consciousness.
  - Prevention of secondary lesions due to cerebral oedema or hypoxia.
- Fracture management
  - Immobilisation of fractures to prevent further damage and relieve pain.
  - Some fractures may require surgery for fixation.
- Other specific interventions
  - The management of other injuries, such as abdominal or pelvic trauma, burns or thermal trauma, depends on the nature and severity of each injury.
- Post-trauma monitoring
  - Patients with polytrauma require close monitoring in an intensive care unit or trauma unit.
  - Pain management, monitoring of vital signs, prevention of complications and regular reassessment are essential.
- Refurbishment
  - Once stabilised, patients often need physical and occupational rehabilitation or other therapies to recover fully or adapt to new limitations.
- Psychosocial support

- Taking into account the psychological impact of a polytrauma is crucial. Patients may need psychological care or support to deal with the emotional after-effects.

The management of polytrauma requires a multidisciplinary approach, combining clinical expertise, responsiveness and coordination between different specialists to ensure the best possible care.

• Craniocerebral trauma

Craniocerebral trauma (CCT) refers to an injury to the brain resulting from external trauma, whether a direct impact to the head or a shearing force following a rapid jolt. They range from mild concussion to severe brain injuries and can have lifelong consequences. Understanding severity, assessment and management is essential for any healthcare professional, particularly in an emergency environment.

- Etiology and mechanism
  - **Common causes**: Road accidents, falls, acts of violence, sports accidents.
  - **Mechanisms**: Direct contusion, blow and counter-blow, shear injuries (axonal diffusion).
- Classification
  - **Mild**: Also known as concussion. Often no loss of consciousness or a brief loss of consciousness.
  - **Moderate**: Loss of consciousness for a few minutes to a few hours, confusion possible for several days or weeks.
  - **Serious**: prolonged loss of consciousness or amnesia, high risk of complications.
- Symptoms and clinical signs
  - Headaches, dizziness, nausea.

- Impaired vision, sensitivity to light or noise.
- Difficulties with concentration or memory.
- Changes in mood or behaviour.
- Assessment and diagnostics
  - **Initial assessment ABCDE**: As with all trauma patients, initial stabilisation is essential.
  - **Glasgow Coma Scale (GCS)**: A standard tool for assessing the level of consciousness.
  - **Imaging**: Brain scan to identify haemorrhages, fractures or other lesions.
- Initial treatment
  - Stabilisation of the airways, breathing and circulation.
  - Cervical immobilisation in cases of suspected cervical spine injury.
  - Reduction of cerebral oedema with drugs such as mannitols.
  - Strict neurological monitoring.
- Possible complications
  - Intracranial haematomas: epidural, subdural, intraparenchymal.
  - Cerebral oedema.
  - Infections if the skull is open or fractured.
  - Seizures.
- Rehabilitation and monitoring
  - Ongoing neurological assessment.
  - Physiotherapy, speech therapy and occupational therapy.
  - Counselling or therapy for emotional or behavioural disorders.
  - Patient and family education on signs of complications or deterioration.
- Prevention
  - Wear helmets when taking part in high-risk sports or activities.
  - Road safety measures.
  - Preventing falls, especially among the elderly.

The management of TBI requires in-depth clinical vigilance and expertise. While many recover fully from mild concussion, severe TBI can have long-term repercussions, requiring multidisciplinary management to optimise recovery.

Acute medical conditions

• Myocardial infarction

A myocardial infarction, commonly known as a heart attack, results from an interruption in the blood supply to part of the heart muscle, leading to ischaemia and tissue necrosis. This acute medical condition is a major cause of morbidity and mortality worldwide. Rapid treatment and accurate diagnosis are essential to optimise patient outcomes.

- Etiology and pathophysiology
    - **Common causes**: Occlusion of a coronary artery by a clot, often following the rupture of an atherosclerotic plaque.
    - **Ischaemia and necrosis**: Loss of oxygen supply causing cell damage and then death of myocardial cells.
- Clinical presentation
    - Chest pain, often described as pressure or crushing.
    - Pain radiates to the left arm, jaw, back or shoulder.
    - Shortness of breath, sweating, nausea, dizziness.
- Diagnosis
    - **Electrocardiogram (ECG)**: Reveals abnormalities specific to ischaemia or infarction.

- **Blood tests**: Increase in cardiac enzymes such as troponin.
  - **Other investigations**: Echocardiography, coronary angiography.
- Initial treatment
  - **Drug treatment**: Aspirin, nitrates, beta-blockers, anticoagulants.
  - **Reperfusion**: Thrombolysis or primary angioplasty to restore blood flow.
- Long-term management
  - Medications : Statins, ACE inhibitors, antiplatelet agents.
  - Lifestyle changes: balanced d i e t , stopping smoking, physical exercise.
  - Cardiac rehabilitation: Supervised programme to improve cardiorespiratory capacity and reduce risk factors.
- Complications
  - Heart failure: Inability of the heart to pump efficiently.
  - Arrhythmias: Abnormal heart rhythms, which can be fatal.
  - Cardiac rupture: rupture of the heart muscle or wall.
- Prevention
  - Controlling risk factors: high blood pressure, high cholesterol, diabetes.
  - Public education: Recognising symptoms and intervening quickly.
- Emotional and psychosocial support
  - Support to deal with anxiety, depression or post-traumatic stress that can occur after a heart attack.
  - Advice for patients and families on returning to a normal life, including resuming physical activity and intimate relationships.

Myocardial infarction is a medical emergency requiring rapid and effective intervention. Prevention, early detection and comprehensive management are essential to improve patients' quality of life and reduce the risk of future complications.

• AVC

Stroke, commonly known as cerebrovascular accident, occurs when the blood supply to part of the brain is interrupted, causing ischaemia of nerve cells that can lead to rapid loss of brain function. Stroke is a medical emergency, and prompt treatment can significantly reduce brain damage and complications.

- Etiology and pathophysiology
    - **Ischaemic stroke**: Caused by occlusion of a cerebral artery. This is the most common type.
    - **Haemorrhagic stroke**: results from the rupture of a blood vessel in the brain.
    - **Risk factors**: Hypertension, smoking, atherosclerosis, atrial fibrillation.
- Clinical presentation
    - Weakness or paralysis on one side of the body.
    - Difficulty speaking or understanding.
    - Impaired vision.
    - Loss of balance or coordination.
    - Sudden, intense headache.
- Diagnosis
    - **Initial assessment**: FAST (Face, Arm, Speech, Time) for rapid assessment.
    - **Imaging**: Computed tomography (CT) or MRI of the brain.
    - **Other investigations**: ECG, carotid ultrasound.

- Initial treatment
  - **For ischaemic stroke**: thrombolysis, anticoagulants.
  - **For haemorrhagic stroke**: control of blood pressure, possible surgery to relieve intracranial pressure.
- Rehabilitation and recovery
  - Physiotherapy to improve mobility and strength.
  - Occupational therapy to regain independence in daily activities.
  - Speech therapy for language disorders.
- Complications
  - Muscular atrophy.
  - Swallowing problems.
  - Post-stroke depression.
- Secondary prevention
  - Control of risk factors: antihypertensive medication, statins.
  - Surgery: such as carotid endarterectomy for certain stenoses.
  - Patient education: diet, exercise, stopping smoking.
- Psychological support
  - Helping patients and their families adapt to life changes.
  - Support groups for patients and carers.
- Getting back to everyday life
  - Advice on resuming driving, work and social activities.
  - Raising awareness of the importance of ongoing medical surveillance.

Stroke is a condition that can profoundly affect the lives of patients and their families. Early treatment, comprehensive rehabilitation and ongoing support can help maximise recovery and improve quality of life after a stroke. Prevention is key, and it is essential to raise public awareness of the warning signs and the importance of seeking help quickly if symptoms arise.

• Asthma attacks

Asthma is a chronic disease of the airways characterised by inflammation and constriction of the bronchial tubes, leading to recurrent episodes of breathlessness, wheezing, coughing and chest tightness. These symptoms can vary in intensity and, in severe cases, can lead to a potentially fatal asthma attack.

- Etiology and pathophysiology
    - **Common triggers** : Allergens, respiratory infections, exercise, cold air, stress.
    - **Inflammatory reaction**: Release of chemical mediators causing oedema, mucus production and bronchial constriction.
- Clinical presentation
    - Shortness of breath.
    - Wheezing on exhalation.
    - Cough, often nocturnal.
    - Feeling of tightness in the chest.
- Diagnosis
    - **Medical history**: frequency, duration, triggers.
    - Functional respiratory investigation (FRI): Measurement of the volume of air inspired and exhaled.
    - **Reversibility test**: Measurement of improvement with a bronchodilator.
- Initial crisis management
    - Rapid-acting bronchodilators: Such as salbutamol.
    - **Oxygen**: If oxygen saturation is low.
    - **Systemic corticosteroids**: To reduce inflammation in severe cases.

- **Monitoring**: Regular assessment of vital signs, work of breathing and oxygen saturation.
- Long-term treatment
  - Long-acting bronchodilators: Such as formoterol.
  - **Inhaled anti-inflammatories:** such as corticosteroids.
  - **Avoiding triggers**: Controlling allergens, stopping smoking.
- Complications
  - Asthmatic status: Severe asthma attack not responding to initial treatment.
  - Respiratory failure.
- Prevention
  - Asthma action plan: Establishment of a written plan to recognise and treat an early exacerbation.
  - Vaccinations: Like the flu vaccine.
  - Education: inhalation techniques, recognising symptoms.
- Psychosocial support
  - Managing the anxiety and stress associated with asthma.
  - Support groups for patients and their families.
- Importance of self-monitoring
  - Using a peak flow meter to monitor lung function at home.
  - Symptom diary to identify and avoid triggers.

An asthma attack is a medical emergency requiring rapid intervention. Understanding and managing the disease are essential to prevent exacerbations, improve quality of life and reduce the risk of complications. Patient education and a strong partnership between patient and healthcare professional are key to successful management.

Chapter 5:
COMMUNICATION IN AN EMERGENCY

Working together
with the medical team

• Working with doctors

In an environment as complex and dynamic as that of the emergency department, close collaboration between nurses and doctors is essential. Effective teamwork can significantly improve patient care, safety and quality of care, while contributing to a harmonious working environment.

- Understanding the respective roles
  - **Nurses**: clinical monitoring, medication administration, patient education, care coordination.
  - **Doctors**: Diagnosis, therapeutic decisions, invasive procedures.
- Effective communication
  - **SBAR (Situation, Background, Assessment, Recommendation)**: A structured tool to facilitate the transmission of information.
  - **Active listening**: Understanding the other person's perspective, asking questions and clarifying doubts.
- Collective decision
  - **Consultation**: Discussing complex care plans or uncertain cases.
  - **Constructive exchanges**: Contribute ideas based on each other's experience and knowledge.

44

- Mutual respect
  - **Recognising expertise**: Valuing the unique contribution of each professional.
  - **Conflict management**: tackling disagreements openly and seeking joint solutions.
- Joint continuing education
  - **Clinical sessions**: Case presentations, updates on emerging practices.
  - **Simulations**: training for emergency situations, reinforcing collaboration.
- Incident support
  - **Debriefings**: Discussing difficult cases or adverse events.
  - **Emotional support**: Recognising stress and exhaustion, offering a listening ear.
- Distribution of responsibilities
  - **Delegation**: knowing when and how to delegate certain tasks or responsibilities.
  - **Nurse autonomy**: Recognising and supporting nurses' skills and decision-making.
- Interdisciplinary
  - **Collaboration with other professionals**: pharmacists, social workers, physiotherapists, etc.
  - **Multidisciplinary meetings**: Promoting a holistic view of the patient.

Working in synergy with doctors is a fundamental pillar of optimal care in the emergency environment. This requires transparent communication, mutual respect and a shared willingness to learn from each other. By cultivating these relationships, nurses and doctors can not only improve the care provided, but also enrich their own professional experience.

• Synergy with other nurses

In an environment as hectic and unpredictable as the emergency department, cohesion and collaboration between nurses are essential. This synergy enhances the quality of care, optimises resources and creates a working atmosphere where every member feels valued and supported.

- Complementary skills
  - **Recognise individual strengths**: Some nurses may have specialist skills or experience.
  - **Learn from each other**: benefit from the knowledge and tips shared by more experienced colleagues.
- Open and transparent communication
  - **Regular exchanges**: sharing information about patients, changes to protocols or challenges encountered.
  - **Constructive feedback**: Encouraging a culture of feedback for continuous improvement.
- Mutual support
  - **Cover during breaks**: Monitoring colleagues' patients during their rest periods.
  - **Helping out during busy periods**: spontaneously coming to the aid of an overworked colleague.
- Planning and coordination
  - **Distribution of tasks**: Divide responsibilities according to skills, preferences and number of patients.
  - **Care transitions**: Ensuring a clear handover during team changes.
- Professional development
  - **Group training**: Organising joint learning sessions.

- **Mentoring**: Experienced nurses can guide and advise newcomers.
- Conflict management
  - **Proactive resolution**: Handling disagreements openly and respectfully.
  - **Mediation**: Using a third party, such as a team leader, to help resolve conflicts.
- Celebrating success
  - **Mutual recognition**: Complimenting a colleague on a job well done.
  - **Team events**: Organise moments of relaxation to strengthen cohesion.
- Well-being and emotional support
  - **Sharing emotions**: Discussing difficult cases or stressful events.
  - **Mutual encouragement**: Supporting each other through difficult times, reminding each other of the importance of looking after ourselves.

Synergy between nurses not only enhances the quality of care, but also professional satisfaction for everyone involved. In the hustle and bustle of emergency care, this solidarity is the glue that keeps the team together, efficient and resilient.

Communicating with patients and families

• Compassion in the face of pain

Pain, whether physical, emotional or psychological, is a universal and profoundly human experience. In the emergency context, where patients often arrive in situations of acute distress, compassion is a cornerstone of nursing care. It transcends the simple medical act to touch the essence of the patient's humanity.

- Understanding pain
  - **The complexity of pain**: Recognising that pain is subjective and can be influenced by physiological, psychological and social factors.
  - **Types of pain**: Differentiate between acute, chronic, neuropathic, somatic, etc. pain.
- Listening and validation
  - **Attentive presence**: Giving the patient your undivided attention when they express their pain.
  - **Validating feelings** : Acknowledging and validating the patient's experience without judgement.
- Holistic pain assessment
  - **Pain scales**: Use standardised tools to assess pain intensity.
  - **Search for underlying causes**: Understanding triggering or aggravating factors.
- Pain management interventions
  - **Pharmacological interventions**: analgesic, anti-inflammatory and adjuvant drugs.
  - **Non-pharmacological interventions**: relaxation techniques, distraction, manual therapies.
- The role of empathy
  - **Put yourself in the patient's shoes**: Imagine what the patient is feeling so that you can adapt your response.
  - **Avoiding compassion burnout**: Becoming aware of your own emotions and knowing when to ask for help.

- Therapeutic communication
  - **Interview techniques**: asking open-ended questions, rephrasing, using touch appropriately.
  - **Managing strong emotions**: Offer support when the patient expresses anger, frustration or fear.
- The spiritual and cultural dimension of pain
  - **Respect for beliefs**: Understanding how culture or spirituality can influence the perception of pain.
  - **Adapting care**: taking account of patients' preferences and beliefs when providing care.
- Self-care and resilience
  - **Recognising the signs of exhaustion**: fatigue, irritability, detachment.
  - **Preservation strategies**: relaxation techniques, supervision, sharing experiences with colleagues.

Compassion in the face of pain is a delicate balance between the desire to provide relief and the ability to remain emotionally stable. For emergency nurses, the ability to respond compassionately to pain is essential to providing quality care while preserving their own well-being.

• Managing the anxiety of loved ones

The anguish felt by relatives when they accompany a patient to emergency is palpable and understandable. Faced with uncertainty, fear and often helplessness, these emotions can interfere with the patient's care and the well-being of the healthcare team. Managing this anxiety is essential not only for the comfort of loved ones, but also for the smooth running of care.

- Recognition and validation
  - **A warm welcome**: A soothing first impression can defuse many anxieties.
  - **Validating emotions**: Recognising and accepting the feelings of loved ones without judgement.
- Transparent communication
  - **Regular updates**: Inform family and friends of the stages in the care process, even if nothing significant has changed.
  - **Active listening**: Giving loved ones the opportunity to express their concerns and questions.
- Education and information
  - **Simple, clear explanations**: Use accessible language to explain procedures or the patient's condition.
  - **Written material**: Provide brochures or information leaflets on current procedures or the pathologies in question.
- Dedicated space
  - **Comfortable waiting room**: A peaceful environment can reduce anxiety.
  - **Rest rooms**: Provide areas to rest, recharge your batteries or take a break from the noise and bustle.

- Dedicated professionals
  - **Social workers**: To offer psychosocial support or adapted resources.
  - **Psychologists**: intervening in particularly traumatic situations.
- Managing conflict situations
  - **De-escalation techniques**: Approach tense situations calmly and assertively.
  - **Security protocols**: Knowing when and how to call in security or the forces of law and order.

- Involvement in care
  - **Participation in care**: Enabling relatives to participate, where possible, in the patient's basic care or comfort.
  - **Support in decision-making**: Involve family members in discussions about therapeutic choices.
- Preparing for discharge or transfer
  - **Clear explanations**: Inform those close to you of the next steps, whether this involves a transfer, hospitalisation or discharge.
  - **Coordination with other departments**: Ensuring a smooth transition to other departments or institutions.

Managing the anxiety of relatives requires a combination of communication skills, empathy and technical knowledge. The challenge for nurses is to find this balance, to ensure that relatives feel supported and informed, while preserving the quality and effectiveness of the care provided to the patient.

Chapter 6:
MANAGING STRESS
AND AVOID BURNOUT

Understanding sources of stress in emergency departments

The emergency department is a particularly intense environment, where decisions often have to be taken quickly and situations can change in an instant. Understanding the sources of stress specific to this environment is essential if we are to manage them more effectively and safeguard the well-being of healthcare professionals.

- Influx of patients
    - **Activity peaks**: Certain periods, such as weekends or holidays, can see a massive influx of patients.
    - **Long   waits**: The pressure of full waiting rooms and long waits can be exhausting.
- Severity of cases
    - **Critical situations**: Treating patients in life-and-death situations puts staff on constant alert.
    - **Decisions with far-reaching consequences**: Every decision, especially in the case of critical patients, can have far-reaching implications.
- Complexity   of cases
    - **Poli-pathological patients**: Managing several medical problems at the same time requires extra vigilance.

- **Lack of history**: Lack of knowledge about a patient's medical history can complicate diagnosis and treatment.
- Emotional factors
    - **Relations with patients and their families**: The emotions of relatives, fear, anxiety or anger can affect staff.
    - **Traumatic situations**: Witnessing suffering, death or tragic events has an emotional impact.
- Logistical pressures
    - **Lack of resources**: A shortage of equipment, beds or staff can increase pressure.
    - **Rapid turnover**: The need to free up beds quickly to accommodate new patients.
- Cross-industry relations
    - **Collaboration with different specialists**: The need to coordinate with other departments or specialist doctors.
    - **Team dynamics**: Tensions or disagreements within the team can be sources of stress.
- Work-life balance
    - **Irregular working hours**: Night shifts, long hours or on-call duty can disrupt personal life.
    - **Mental workload**: Bringing work home, whether physically or emotionally.
- Physical environment
    - **Noise and commotion**: The constant coming and going, the alarms and the general commotion can be trying.
    - **Physical demands**: Standing for long periods, lifting patients, repetitive movements.

Understanding these sources of stress is the first step in developing management and resilience strategies. By recognising the specific challenges of the emergency department, healthcare professionals can better prepare, adapt and seek the support they need to maintain a healthy and sustainable practice.

Relaxation techniques and decompression

After hours spent managing emergency situations, nurses can feel a high level of physical and mental tension. Learning to relax and decompress is essential to maintaining your well-being and your ability to provide quality care. Here are some effective techniques and methods for promoting relaxation and decompression:

- Deep breathing
    - **4-7-8 technique**: Inhale through your nose for 4 seconds, hold your breath for 7 seconds, then exhale through your mouth for 8 seconds. This method is excellent for calming the mind quickly.
    - **Abdominal breathing**: Concentrate on breathing with your abdomen rather than your chest for maximum relaxation.
- Meditation and mindfulness
    - **Guided meditation**: Use applications or recordings to follow a meditation session.
    - **Full awareness**: Be present in the moment, observe your sensations and thoughts, without judgement.
- Physical exercise
    - **Yoga**: The postures and breathing of yoga can help release muscular tension and calm the mind.
    - **Brisk walking or jogging**: Cardiovascular exercise releases endorphins, which are powerful natural painkillers.

54

- Visualisation techniques
  - **Guided visualisation**: Imagine yourself in a peaceful place, such as a beach or a forest, to escape the hustle and bustle of the moment.
  - **Positive visualisation**: Focus on positive outcomes and happy scenarios to lift your mood.
- Progressive muscle relaxation
  - Learn to tense and release each muscle group, starting with the toes and working up to the head.
- Reflective writing
  - **Gratitude diary**: Write down three things each day for which you are grateful.
  - **Decompression diary**: Write down your experiences, feelings and thoughts to externalise them.
- Listening to music
  - Choose soothing melodies or nature sounds to help you relax. The music you love can also lift your spirits.
- Self-massage techniques
  - **Temple massage**: Ideal for relieving headaches.
  - **Hand and wrist massage**: Useful for nurses who perform repetitive manual tasks.
- Regular breaks
  - Take short breaks to stretch your body, close your eyes or simply breathe deeply.
- Hot baths and showers
- The warmth relaxes the muscles and provides a feeling of well-being.
- Alternative therapies
- **Acupuncture**: Can help relieve stress and tension.
- **Aromatherapy**: Using essential oils such as lavender or chamomile can have a soothing effect.

The important thing is to recognise when you need to decompress and to take the time to do so. Incorporating these techniques into your daily routine can help prevent burn-out and improve your quality of life both at work and outside.

Supervision and support among colleagues

The emergency department is an environment where stressful and unpredictable situations are commonplace. In this context, supervision and support between colleagues are crucial to guaranteeing quality patient care while preserving the mental and emotional health of carers.

- The importance of supervision:
    - **Continuous learning**: Supervision enables less experienced nurses to benefit from the knowledge and expertise of their more experienced colleagues.
    - **Improving practice**: Supervision enables carers to adjust and improve their techniques and clinical approaches.
    - **Error prevention**: A second pair of eyes or a second opinion can help prevent medical errors.
- The value of mutual support:
    - **Shared emotions**: Sharing difficult situations with others means you don't have to carry the weight of your emotions and responsibilities alone.
    - **Practical advice**: Colleagues can offer tips or techniques that have been tried and tested in similar situations.

- **Team cohesion**: Supporting each other strengthens team solidarity and encourages better collaboration.
- Supervision arrangements:
  - **Regular meetings**: Organise dedicated times to discuss practices, complex cases and difficulties encountered.
  - **Real-time observation**: Experienced nurses can observe and advise their colleagues as they perform technical procedures.
- Create an environment of trust:
  - **Open communication**: Encourage team members to share their concerns and questions without fear of judgement.
  - **Mutual respect**: Valuing the contribution of each team member, whatever their level of experience.
- Emotional support strategies:
  - **Discussion groups**: Organise sessions where the team can talk about their feelings and emotions.
  - **Active listening**: Learning to listen to colleagues without interrupting them, and giving them space to express themselves.
- Continuing education:
  - **Workshops**: Organising workshops to share best practice and the latest advances in emergency care.
  - **Constructive feedback**: Providing kind and constructive feedback to enable everyone to progress.
- Team well-being:
  - **Relaxation activities**: Organise activities outside work to strengthen team cohesion and allow everyone to unwind.

- **Raising awareness of burn-out**: Being alert to signs of fatigue and burn-out, and encouraging dialogue on the subject.

Supervision and support between colleagues are essential to guaranteeing the quality of care while preserving the well-being of carers. In a demanding environment like emergency care, looking after each other is not just beneficial, it's vital.

Chapter 7:
ETHICS AND PROFESSIONAL CONDUCT

The principles of medical ethics

Medical ethics guide the behaviour of healthcare professionals in their day-to-day practice. These principles aim to ensure quality care, respect for the patient and human dignity. Emergencies, with their unpredictable nature and fast pace, can test the medical team's adherence to these principles. Nevertheless, it is essential to respect them in order to preserve trust between carers and patients.

- Principle of autonomy:
    - **Respect for patient choice**: Patients have the right to decide on their treatment after being properly informed.
    - **Informed consent**: Before any intervention or treatment, it is essential to ensure that the patient has fully understood and accepted the implications.
- The principle of beneficence:
    - **Acting in the patient's best interests**: Every action or decision must be taken in the patient's best interests to improve his or her condition or well-being.
    - **Health promotion**: In addition to emergency care, patients should be advised on the best practices for their long-term health.
- The principle of non-maleficence:
    - **Do no harm**: It is vital to avoid causing damage or harm to the patient, even in the course of treatment.

- **Risk-benefit assessment**: Before any intervention, it is necessary to weigh up the potential benefits against the associated risks.
- Principle of justice:
  - **Fair treatment**: Every patient is entitled to the same level of care, regardless of their social, economic or ethnic situation.
  - **Limited resources**: In an emergency context, where resources may be limited, it is essential to distribute them fairly.
- Confidentiality:
  - **Data protection**: All information relating to the patient must be kept confidential, except in very specific circumstances.
  - **Sharing information**: Communication between healthcare professionals concerning a patient must respect the patient's privacy.
- Honesty and truth:
  - **Transparency**: Patients must be given clear and honest information about their condition, treatment options, risks and prognosis.
  - **Acknowledging errors**: If an error is made, it is the responsibility of the healthcare professional to admit it and inform the patient.
- Professionalism:
  - **Ongoing training**: Healthcare professionals must continually update their knowledge and skills.
  - **Limits of competence**: It is crucial to recognise one's own limits and to ask for help or redirect the patient if necessary.
- Respect for the individual:
  - **Human dignity**: Every patient, regardless of their condition or circumstances, deserves respect, empathy and consideration.

- **Cultural sensitivity**: It is important to take account of each patient's beliefs, values and customs.

Medical practice in emergency departments is complex, but these ethical principles provide a solid framework for navigating through the challenges and ensuring that every decision is taken in the best interests of the patient.

Common emergency room dilemmas

• End of life and palliative care

In an emergency department, professionals are often confronted with life and death situations, and sometimes with the management of terminally ill or dying patients. Although the main focus of the emergency department is on stabilising and saving life, it is essential to understand and integrate the philosophy of palliative care into the management of these patients.

- Understanding the end of life:
  - **Definition**: What is the end of life? Recognising the signs and symptoms that indicate a patient is terminally ill.
  - **Acceptance**: For staff, accepting the finitude of life can be a challenge, but it is essential if they are to offer appropriate care.
- Palliative care:
  - **Definition and objectives**: Palliative care aims to improve the quality of life of patients and their families in the face of the consequences of a life-threatening illness.
  - **Pain control**: Pain management is central to palliative care, to ensure that patients are as comfortable as possible.

- Communication with patients and families:
  - **Delivering the bad news**: How to deal with a serious diagnosis or an unfavourable outcome with empathy and compassion.
  - **Emotional support**: Providing a space for patients and their families to express their feelings, fears and concerns.
- Medical decisions at the end of life:
  - **Advance directives**: understanding the patient's wishes regarding treatment and interventions at the end of life.
  - **Non-resuscitation**: Discussing and respecting the patient's choice not to intervene in the event of cardiac or respiratory arrest.
- Ethical aspects:
  - **Respecting the patient's wishes**: Even in an emergency situation, it is essential to take account of the patient's end-of-life wishes.
  - **Limiting and stopping treatments**: Knowing when and how to limit or stop treatments that are no longer beneficial.
- Psychological support:
  - **Anticipated grievance**: Recognising and supporting the emotions of loved ones who are experiencing bereavement even before the patient dies.
  - **Post-mortem bereavement**: Providing resources and support to the family after the death of a loved one.
- Support for care staff:
  - **Dealing with emotional exhaustion**: Emergencies can be stressful, especially when dealing with deaths. Finding ways to deal with stress and grief is crucial.
  - **Supervision and debriefing**: Providing opportunities to discuss difficult cases and the associated emotions.

- Working with the palliative care team:
  - **Consultation**: Seek the expertise of the palliative care team to ensure optimal care.
  - **Continuing education**: Regular training in the principles of palliative care and how to integrate them into the emergency context.

Caring for patients at the end of life in an emergency department requires a multidimensional, patient-centred approach that combines medical, ethical and interpersonal skills. By integrating the principles of palliative care, emergency staff can offer respectful, dignified and compassionate care to these patients and their families.

• Dealing with cases of violence or abuse

In an emergency department, nurses may be confronted with patients who have been victims of violence or abuse. This is a delicate situation, requiring a specific medical, psychological and social approach. The aim is to protect the patient, treat their injuries and direct them to the appropriate resources.

- Recognising signs of violence or abuse:
  - **Physical signs**: Injuries, bruises, fractures, burns, which may indicate physical abuse.
  - **Psychological signs**: Anxiety, depression, behavioural changes, sleep disorders, which may indicate emotional or psychological abuse.
  - **Signs of sexual abuse**: genital trauma, sexually transmitted infections, age-inappropriate sexual behaviour.
- Initial approach:
  - **Creating a safe environment**: Ensuring confidentiality and privacy for the patient.

- **Listen sympathetically**: Letting patients express themselves without pressure, judgement or prejudice.
- Medical assessment:
  - **Complete physical examination**: Identify and document all injuries.
  - **Additional examinations**: X-rays, blood tests, samples taken in cases of suspected sexual abuse.
- Psychological care:
  - **Assessment of psychological distress**: To determine the level of post-traumatic stress, anxiety or depression.
  - **Referral to a psychologist or psychiatrist**: For specialist treatment if necessary.
- Patient protection:
  - **Reporting**: If abuse is confirmed or strongly suspected, it may be necessary to report it to the relevant authorities.
  - **Safety**: If the patient is in danger, consider sheltering or hospitalisation.
- Social support:
  - **Referral to specialist associations**: These can offer legal, psychological and social support.
  - **Assistance with administrative formalities**: filing a complaint, legal proceedings, etc.
- Long-term care:
  - **Regular medical follow-up**: To treat the physical and psychological after-effects.
  - **Specific therapies**: Psychotherapy, discussion groups, to help the patient overcome the trauma.
- Training and prevention:
  - **Raising staff awareness**: Regular training for emergency staff on how to recognise and deal with violence and abuse.

- **Prevention campaigns**: Participating in awareness campaigns to prevent violence and abuse in the community.

Treating patients who are victims of violence or abuse in emergency departments is a major challenge that requires a comprehensive, multidisciplinary approach. It requires not only medical skills, but also great sensitivity, active listening and close collaboration with other professionals and specialist organisations.

Chapter 8:
THE TECHNOLOGY
IN THE EMERGENCY DEPARTMENT

Advanced diagnostic tools

• Point-of-care ultrasound

Point-of-care ultrasound (POCUS) has become an invaluable tool in the management of patients in the emergency department. It allows nurses and doctors to visualise a patient's internal organs and structures in real time, offering an unrivalled diagnostic advantage for certain conditions.

- Introduction to POCUS:
    - **Definition**: Understanding what POCUS is and how it differs from traditional ultrasound scans.
    - **Benefits**: Speed, non-invasiveness, bedside use, improved clinical decision-making.
- Technical basics:
    - **Ultrasound principles**: How ultrasound works and its underlying principles.
    - **Handling the probe**: Basic techniques for obtaining a good image.
    - **Image interpretation**: Recognition of normal and pathological structures.
- Current clinical applications:
    - **Cardiac assessment**: Visualisation of the heart to detect abnormalities such as tamponade or hypovolaemia.
    - **Pulmonary assessment**: look for effusions, pneumothorax or signs of acute pulmonary oedema.

- **Traumatology**: Rapid assessment of internal bleeding, particularly in the context of abdominal or thoracic trauma.
- **Abdominal assessment**: Detection of ascites, assessment of the gall bladder, kidneys or abdominal aorta.
- **Vessel assessment**: Identification of deep vein thrombosis or assessment of circulation status.
- Limitations and pitfalls:
  - **Recognition of artefacts**: Understanding images that may be misleading or misinterpreted.
  - **Limitations of the examination**: Know when POCUS is not the appropriate tool and when other imaging modalities are required.
- Integration of POCUS into the emergency department workflow:
  - **When to use POCUS**: Identify situations where POCUS is particularly useful.
  - **Documentation and archiving**: Ensuring appropriate follow-up of results and interpretations.
- Training and certification:
  - **Training programmes**: Where and how to obtain training in POCUS for emergencies.
  - **Certification and skills**: Understanding the standards and requirements for practising POCUS competently.
- Ethics and legality:
  - **Patient consent**: Ensure that patients understand and consent to the examination.
  - **Legal risks**: Understanding the implications of misinterpretation or misdiagnosis.

The integration of POCUS into the emergency department has revolutionised the way healthcare professionals assess and treat patients. It provides a real-time view of a patient's internal condition, which is crucial in an environment where every second counts. With the right training and judicious use, POCUS can dramatically improve emergency care.

• Cardiac monitors and telecardiology

Cardiac monitoring and telecardiology are essential tools in the medical world, making it possible to assess patients' cardiac condition in real time and provide rapid and appropriate intervention, even at a distance. Emergency departments, in particular, benefit from these technologies for the management of patients suffering from cardiac disorders.

- Introduction to cardiac monitors:
    - **What is a cardiac monitor**: Understanding the basic principles of cardiac monitoring.
    - **Monitoring objectives**: Detect arrhythmias, assess cardiac function, monitor after an operation or treatment.
- Cardiac monitor technologies:
    - **Electrocardiography (ECG)**: Monitoring the electrical activity of the heart to detect irregularities.
    - **Pulse oximetry**: Measurement of oxygen saturation in the blood.
    - **Non-invasive blood pressure (NIBP)**: Monitoring of blood pressure at regular intervals.
- Data interpretation:
    - **Reading an ECG**: Identifying the different waves and understanding their meaning.
    - **Detecting arrhythmias**: Recognising normal and abnormal rhythms.
    - **Responding to alarms**: Understanding alert thresholds and knowing how to intervene.

- Introduction to telecardiology:
  - **Definition and challenges**: Using communication technologies to provide remote cardiac care.
  - **Applications**: Remote monitoring, remote ECG interpretation, virtual consultations with cardiologists.
- Advantages of telecardiology:
  - **Greater access to specialists**: For patients in remote or underserved areas.
  - **Rapid response**: Reduced waiting time for an interpretation or intervention.
  - **Continuous monitoring**: Patients can be monitored at home, reducing the need for prolonged hospital stays.
- Challenges and concerns:
  - **Reliability of the technology**: Ensuring stable and secure data transmission.
  - **Training**: Ensure that staff are trained in the use of these tools and can integrate them effectively into their care.
- Ethics and confidentiality:
  - **Data protection**: guaranteeing the security of patients' medical information.
  - **Informed consent**: Ensuring patients understand and consent to telemonitoring.
- The future of telecardiology:
  - **Technological innovations**: Looking ahead to future developments that could transform the way we monitor and treat patients.
  - **Expansion of services**: Consider how telecardiology could be extended to other medical fields.

The combination of cardiac monitoring and telecardiology offers an exceptional opportunity to improve the quality of cardiac care. In an increasingly connected world, these tools enable healthcare professionals to be in constant touch with their patients' hearts, whether they are at their side or miles away.

Telemedicine and emergency services

In today's digital age, telemedicine has become an essential tool for improving the quality and efficiency of medical care. In the emergency context, it offers innovative solutions for responding rapidly to medical crises and optimising resources.

- Introduction to telemedicine:
    - **What is telemedicine**: definition, origins and fundamental principles.
    - **Types of telemedicine**: telemonitoring, teleconsultation, tele-expertise and teleassistance.
- The value of telemedicine in emergencies:
    - **Access to specialists**: real-time connection with experts, even in remote or underserved areas.
    - **Real-time response**: faster diagnosis and decision-making in critical situations.
    - **Optimisation of resources**: Efficient distribution of patients, avoiding unnecessary bottlenecks.
- Implementation of telemedicine in emergency departments:
    - **Equipment required**: Technical infrastructure, software and communications equipment.
    - **Management protocols**: Development of clear procedures for the use of telemedicine.

- **Staff training**: Ensure that the emergency team is competent and comfortable with telemedicine tools.
- Practical examples and case studies:
  - **Cerebrovascular accidents (CVA)**: Use of telemedicine for rapid consultation with a specialist neurologist.
  - **Trauma and injuries**: Remote assessment to determine the level of care required.
  - **Rural and isolated situations**: Link with major medical centres for complex or serious situations.
- Challenges and concerns of telemedicine in emergencies:
  - **Reliability of technology**: Ensuring stable, high-quality communications.
  - **Confidentiality and security**: Protection of medical data and respect for patient privacy.
  - **Legal issues and liability**: Clarification of responsibilities in telemedicine.
- Ethics and telemedicine:
  - **Informed consent**: Ensuring that patients understand and accept teleconsultation.
  - **Quality of care**: Maintaining high standards and ensuring equity of access.
- The future of telemedicine in emergencies:
  - **Technological innovations**: future advances and their impact on emergency departments.
  - **Integration into healthcare systems**: Reflections on how telemedicine could reshape the entire medical landscape.

Emergency departments are, by their very nature, places where every second counts. Telemedicine offers the opportunity to make the most of those precious seconds, connecting patients to healthcare professionals with unprecedented efficiency and speed. As technology continues to evolve, it is essential that emergency professionals are at the forefront of these changes, ensuring the best possible care for those who need it most.

Information systems and patient management

Information systems (IS) have revolutionised the way healthcare establishments manage and process patient data. In an emergency environment, these systems are all the more crucial, offering solutions to optimise patient care, guarantee continuity of care and improve operational efficiency.

- Introduction to information systems:
    - **Definition and role of IS**: Understanding the importance of IS in the modern medical world.
    - **History**: Evolution of IS from paper documentation to advanced digital platforms.
- The benefits of IS in emergency departments:
    - **Quick access to medical records**: instant retrieval of medical history, allergies, current treatments, etc.
    - **Care coordination**: Improved communication between healthcare professionals for integrated care.
    - **Real-time monitoring**: Monitoring of available beds, intervention schedules and medication levels.
- Key components of emergency IS:
    - **Electronic medical records (EMR)**: Digital storage of patient medical information.
    - Admissions, discharges and transfers management systems (ADT): Tracking the patient's journey through the hospital.

- **Triage and assessment tools**: Help in prioritising cases according to severity.
- Interconnectivity and integration:
  - **Interoperability**: The ability of systems to exchange and use information transparently.
  - **Integration with other departments**: Facilitating communication with radiology, laboratories, etc.
  - **Connection with other establishments**: information sharing for transfers or specialist consultations.
- Security and confidentiality:
  - **Data protection**: Measures to secure sensitive information.
  - **Patient confidentiality**: Ensuring compliance with privacy and medical data regulations.
  - **Backup and recovery**: Protocols in the event of system failure or disaster.
- Staff training and adaptation:
  - **Ongoing training**: Ensuring that the team is up to date with new features and updates.
  - **Technology adoption**: Overcoming resistance and encouraging optimum use of IS.
  - **Technical support**: Help is available if you have any problems or questions.
- The future of IS in emergency departments:
  - **Artificial intelligence and predictive analysis**: Predicting trends, such as patient influxes, using historical data.
  - **Integrated telemedicine**: Direct connection with remote specialists via the IS.
  - **Patient portals**: Enabling patients to access their own medical information and communicate with medical staff.

Information systems are therefore the beating heart of modern emergency services, playing a crucial role in the coordination, efficiency and quality of care. By integrating technology into emergency procedures, facilities can ensure faster, safer and more personalised care for every patient.

Chapter 9:
INTERCULTURAL ISSUES
AND DIVERSITY

Understanding and respecting cultural diversity

In an increasingly interconnected world and increasingly diverse societies, emergency departments are often the meeting point of many cultures. Caring for patients from diverse cultural backgrounds requires a deep understanding and genuine respect for their beliefs, practices and needs.

- Cultural diversity: an omnipresent reality:
    - **Defining cultural diversity**: Understanding what "culture" means and how it influences our behaviour and perceptions.
    - **The importance of diversity in the medical context**: How cultural differences can influence the perception of pain, illness and death.
- Challenges related to cultural diversity in emergency departments:
    - **Language barriers:** Communication difficulties and risks of misunderstanding.
    - **Traditional beliefs and medical practices**: How they can conflict with or complement Western medicine.
    - **Concepts of modesty and intimacy**: different standards that can influence patient comfort during physical examinations.

- Strategies for appropriate management:
  - **Intercultural training for staff**: Raising awareness and training staff about different cultures and potential challenges.
  - **Medical interpreters**: their crucial role in facilitating communication.
  - **Multilingual information material**: Ensuring that patients and families understand procedures, rights and responsibilities.
- Respect for religious rites and beliefs:
  - **The importance of the spiritual in medical care**: Understanding the rituals surrounding illness, death and healing.
  - **Practical arrangements**: Adapting medical procedures to comply with religious prohibitions or obligations.
- Taking account of the cultural dimension in medical ethics:
  - **Informed consent**: ensuring that it is given with respect for cultural beliefs.
  - **End of life**: Respecting wishes and beliefs around death and dying.
  - **Relationship with the family**: In some cultures, the family plays a central role in medical decisions.
- Building trust and mutual respect:
  - **Active listening**: Valuing the patient's concerns and needs.
  - **Empathy**: Putting yourself in the patient's shoes to better understand their feelings and concerns.
  - **Feedback**: Regularly solicit feedback to continually improve care.
- The urgent future of cultural diversity:
  - **Demographic trends**: Changing populations and the need to constantly adapt services.

- **Research and case studies**: The importance of studying cultural diversity to optimise management protocols.

Emergency services, by their very nature, must be ready to welcome everyone, without discrimination. Recognising, understanding and respecting cultural diversity is not simply a moral or ethical obligation, it is a necessity for providing quality care and ensuring the safety and well-being of patients. It is by embracing this diversity that healthcare professionals can offer holistic care, characterised by respect and humanity.

Intercultural communication: challenges and techniques

The emergency department, often compared to a gateway to the healthcare system, is a place where healthcare professionals encounter a diversity of patients from different cultural backgrounds. In this context, intercultural communication becomes an essential skill for providing quality care. This chapter aims to explore the challenges associated with intercultural communication and to present techniques for overcoming them.

- Understanding intercultural communication:
    - **What is intercultural communication**: Exploring the concept and its importance in the medical context.
    - **The cultural dimension of communication**: how culture influences the way we communicate, our expectations and our interpretations.

- The major challenges of intercultural communication:
    - **Language barriers**: Mistakes in translation and interpretation can have serious consequences in medicine.
    - **Differences in non-verbal expressions**: Gestures, eye contact and proximity can have different meanings in different cultures.
    - **Differences in value systems and beliefs**: How cultural conceptions of health, illness and medicine influence communication.
- Techniques for improving intercultural communication:
    - **Use medical interpreters**: Not only for literal translation, but also to help navigate cultural nuances.
    - **Active listening**: Show empathy, ask open-ended questions and rephrase to make sure you understand.
    - **Validation**: Ensure that the patient has understood the information provided.
    - **Use of visual material**: Images and diagrams can transcend language barriers.
- Training and awareness-raising:
    - **Training programmes in intercultural communication**: Providing healthcare professionals with the tools to navigate effectively in a multicultural environment.
    - **Case studies**: Analysing real-life situations to learn lessons and improve practices.
- The importance of feedback:
    - **Regular evaluation**: Gathering feedback from patients and families to continually improve communication.
    - **Supervision and support between colleagues**: Sharing experiences, successes and challenges to learn from each other.

- Building an environment conducive to intercultural communication:
  - **Multilingual display**: Ensuring that essential information is available in the main languages spoken by patients.
  - **Encouraging diversity among staff**: Hiring staff from different cultures can facilitate communication and rapport with patients.
- The future of intercultural communication:
  - **Technologies and tools**: The growing use of telemedicine, translation applications and other technological innovations to improve communication.
  - **Research and development**: The importance of intercultural communication research in adapting practices to socio-cultural changes.

Intercultural communication is an essential skill in the modern medical world, particularly in an environment as diverse as emergency departments. It requires careful listening, an open mind and a constant willingness to learn and adapt. Ultimately, effective communication is the foundation of quality medical care, guaranteeing the safety, respect and dignity of every patient.

Specific aspects of care to vulnerable populations

Emergency services play an essential role in the care of vulnerable populations. Whether they are homeless people, refugees, the elderly, children, people with disabilities or other at-risk groups, caring for these patients presents unique challenges and requires special sensitivity and training. This chapter details the specifics of this care.

- Recognising vulnerability:
    - **Definition and types of vulnerability**: Understanding the many facets of vulnerability.
    - **Associated risk factors**: Social, economic, physiological and psychological.
- Vulnerable populations and their specific needs:
    - **Homeless people**: the challenges of access to care, specific health problems and care coordination.
    - **Refugees and asylum seekers**: Trauma, language and cultural barriers, and the importance of holistic care.
    - **The elderly**: frailty, polypathology and the need for a comprehensive assessment.
    - **Children**: Paediatric care, communication challenges and psychosocial needs.
    - **People with disabilities**: adapting care to their needs, ensuring accessibility and appropriate communication.
- Appropriate, empathetic communication:
    - **Specific communication techniques**: Adaptation according to the type of vulnerability.
    - **Establishing trust**: The importance of creating a safe environment for these patients.
- Multidisciplinary approach:
    - **Coordination of care**: Ensuring continuity of care with other departments and specialities.
    - **Networking**: integrating social workers, psychologists and other professionals to provide comprehensive care.
- Medical ethics and vulnerable populations:
    - **Informed consent**: Ensuring that patients understand procedures while respecting their autonomy.
    - **Confidentiality**: Preserving dignity and privacy, especially in vulnerable situations.

- Training to care for vulnerable   populations:
    - **Awareness programmes**: Educating staff about the specific challenges associated with these populations.
    - **Exercises and case studies**: Enabling healthcare professionals to practise in a controlled environment.
- Prevention and guidance strategies:
    - **Early detection**: Identify signs of vulnerability as soon as you arrive at A&E.
    - **Refer patients   to appropriate facilities**: Ensuring appropriate care after discharge from A&E.
- The future of care for vulnerable   populations:
    - **Innovation and best practice**: Investigating and adopting new methods to improve care.
    - **Public health policies**: The importance of a global approach to meet the needs of vulnerable populations.

Caring for vulnerable populations in emergency departments requires a humanistic approach, specific training and close collaboration between different professionals. It is by recognising these specificities and acting proactively that emergency departments can truly meet the needs of these patients and guarantee the quality and dignity of care.

Chapter 10:
DISASTER MANAGEMENT
AND EXCEPTIONAL SITUATIONS

Basic principles disaster medicine

Disaster medicine stands like a beacon in the tumultuous ocean of extreme situations, illuminating the way forward for healthcare professionals when the norm vanishes in the face of the magnitude of the event. Born of the need to respond effectively to major crises, whether caused by natural disasters, acts of terrorism or pandemics, this medical speciality is based on fundamental principles for managing the unexpected.

At the heart of disaster medicine is the concept of triage, a rigorous process for prioritising care. In a context where resources are limited and demand exponential, triage becomes an art. It involves quickly determining which of the injured or sick require immediate care and which can wait, in order to save as many lives as possible. This decision, although difficult, is essential to maximise the effectiveness of the medical response.

But beyond triage, disaster medicine also relies on solid organisation and coordination. Medical teams have to function like a synchronised orchestra, with each member knowing his or her role perfectly, but also being able to adapt to the unexpected. Because that's another characteristic of disaster medicine: uncertainty is a constant, and the ability to adapt becomes an invaluable skill.

Logistics also play a key role. The rapid establishment of emergency medical camps, the supply of equipment and medicines, and coordination with other agencies and organisations all form the foundation on which the medical response is built.

Finally, the psychological aspect must not be neglected. Victims of disasters, as well as those involved, can be profoundly affected by the event. Dealing with psychological trauma, supporting and accompanying individuals, is just as crucial as physical care.

The complexity and importance of disaster medicine is a reminder that in the darkest of times, it is a structured, thoughtful and humane approach that can make the difference and bring a glimmer of hope in the midst of chaos.

Emergencies in crisis situations: Attacks, natural disasters...

Faced with the suddenness and scale of crisis situations, whether attacks or natural disasters, the world of emergency services is plunged into a whirlwind of frenetic activity, reflecting the urgency of the situation. These extraordinary events demand a capacity to adapt and respond rapidly, while preserving the quality and safety of care.

In the chaos of terrorist attacks, with their explosions and multiple victims, or the devastation caused by natural disasters such as earthquakes, floods or hurricanes, emergency services are the first on the front line. The unpredictable nature of these events puts the preparedness, resilience and speed of response of medical teams to the test.

The major challenge for emergency services is managing the large number of victims in a very short space of time. Every second counts, and triage is becoming a central element of care. The seriously injured, requiring immediate intervention, are separated from those whose condition is less critical, thereby maximising the chances of survival for as many as possible.

But beyond immediate medical care, these crisis situations reveal other issues that are just as crucial. Communication, both internally between healthcare professionals and externally with the public, is essential to disseminate clear information, manage expectations and avoid panic. At the same time, coordination with other emergency services, whether local or international, is vital to ensure a coherent and effective response.

The psychological dimension of these crises cannot be underestimated. Victims and their families, as well as those involved, can be deeply affected by the severity and brutality of these events. Offering psychological support, recognising the signs of post-traumatic stress and ensuring long-term follow-up are all key elements in helping everyone to overcome these ordeals.

Ultimately, while these crisis situations highlight the vulnerability of our society in the face of major events, they also reveal the strength, determination and solidarity of medical teams. These professionals, often risking their own lives, strive to provide comfort and care in extreme conditions, embodying the unwavering dedication of the medical vocation.

Preparation and specific training for these situations

Preparing for crisis situations is an ongoing quest, at the crossroads of science, experience and strategy. On the eve of a tragic event, every second, every decision and every action counts, and that's where the inestimable value of specific training for these situations lies.

For healthcare professionals, training is not just about acquiring medical skills. It encompasses a wide range of knowledge which, when combined, forms a holistic and effective approach to crisis management.

Simulation and practical scenarios: Medical simulation is a valuable tool that offers healthcare professionals an opportunity to practise emergency situations in a controlled environment. Using realistic scenarios, they can develop and refine their skills, learn to work as part of a team and make decisions under pressure.

Triage and mass management: Crisis situations often require a large number of casualties to be triaged quickly. Specific training teaches how to effectively assess a person's condition, determine the level of care required and prioritise interventions.

Crisis communication: Medical teams must learn to communicate effectively not only with each other, but also with victims, their families and the media. Clear and effective communication can reduce confusion, fear and chaos.

Stress management and psychological support: Given the seriousness and pressure inherent in these events, it is crucial that emergency responders are trained to recognise and manage their own stress, while offering psychological support to victims.

Specific protocols and equipment: Crisis situations may require the use of specific equipment or protocols, from first aid kits in the event of a chemical attack to special procedures for victims of collapses.

Interdisciplinary collaboration: Crisis situations require a coordinated response involving not only the medical services, but also the emergency services, police, fire brigade and other organisations. Training in interdisciplinary collaboration is therefore essential.

Training for these specific situations is an ongoing commitment. Protocols evolve, new methods emerge and lessons learned from past events shape future approaches. By investing in this training, we are forging a resilient, seasoned force ready to respond, able to stand up to adversity with skill and compassion.

Chapter 11:
CLINICAL RESEARCH
IN EMERGENCIES

The importance of research in emergency settings

Emergency research is not simply an academic branch of medicine; it is the pillar that guides and shapes the way emergency care is delivered, continuously improving the quality, effectiveness and innovation of interventions. This research, by immersing itself in the analysis and study of emergency situations, diseases and treatments, becomes an essential lever for saving more lives and improving patient outcomes.

Understanding for better treatment: Every emergency situation is unique, but patterns and trends can emerge through in-depth study. By documenting and analysing these cases, researchers can develop more effective protocols, refine existing techniques or even discover new therapeutic approaches.

Protocol evaluation: Medical protocols are not set in stone. They need to be continually evaluated and revised. Research provides a framework for testing the effectiveness of these protocols, ensuring that they are based on solid evidence and adapting them to new discoveries or changing contexts.

Technological innovation: Technology is playing an increasingly important role in emergency medicine. Whether through new diagnostic equipment, telemedicine tools or advanced information systems, research is essential to evaluate, improve and integrate these innovations into daily practice.

Training and education: Thanks to research, training for healthcare professionals can be evidence-based, ensuring that nurses and doctors are trained in the most effective and up-to-date techniques.

Responding to major crises: In situations such as pandemics, terrorist attacks or natural disasters, real-time research becomes vital. It enables us to understand the situation, develop appropriate interventions and rapidly share this knowledge with the global medical community.

Promoting medical ethics: Research in emergency settings also helps to define and reaffirm ethical principles in complex situations where decisions have to be taken quickly.

Anticipating future challenges: Emergency medicine, like all medical disciplines, is evolving. Research helps us to anticipate future challenges, whether they be new diseases, demographic changes or societal developments.

Research in emergency medicine is the beacon that lights the way for emergency medicine. It ensures that every action, every decision, every treatment is the fruit of in-depth knowledge, rigorous evaluation and a constant desire to improve and perfect patient care. In the midst of tumult and urgency, it is this research that offers the serenity of informed action.

Taking part in a clinical trial: roles and responsibilities

Taking part in a clinical trial is a crucial step in the development of new drugs, treatments and medical approaches. These trials play a central role in expanding our medical understanding and ensuring that treatments are both safe and effective. But behind the science and the statistics lies a human infrastructure, made up of researchers, patients and many other players, each with well-defined roles and responsibilities.

The researchers :
Responsibilities :
- Design the study by clearly defining the objectives, inclusion and exclusion criteria, and methodology.
- Obtain ethical approval to ensure that the trial complies with ethical and legal standards.
- Monitor the study to ensure that it is proceeding as planned and adjust if necessary.
- Analyse data to draw objective conclusions.

Roles :
- Provide appropriate medical care for participants.
- Inform participants in a clear and transparent manner about the risks, benefits, conduct of the trial and any other relevant information.
- Guarantee the confidentiality of participants' data.

The participants:
Responsibilities :
- Provide accurate information about their health, medical history and any other factors relevant to the study.
- Scrupulously follow the instructions given by the researchers.
- Report any anomalies or side-effects observed.

- Undertake to take part in the study for its entire duration, except in the event of medical contraindication or other valid reasons.

Roles :
- Play an active role by asking questions and trying to understand all aspects of the trial.
- Participate voluntarily, in the knowledge that they can withdraw at any time without suffering any negative consequences.
- Contribute to the advancement of medical science by providing valuable data for the trial.

The ethics committee :
Responsibilities :
- Evaluate the clinical trial to ensure that it is ethically and legally acceptable.
- Monitor the trial to ensure that ethical standards are maintained throughout.
- Intervene if ethical problems are identified.

Roles :
- To act as a guardian of ethical standards in medical research.
- Providing expertise in medical ethics to researchers and participants.

A clinical trial is a complex partnership between researchers, participants and ethics committees. Each player has specific roles and responsibilities which, when respected, ensure the ethical conduct of research and the production of high-quality data that can transform and improve the medical landscape for all.

Recent advances
thanks to emergency research

Emergency medicine, as a dynamic and constantly evolving field, has seen many advances in recent years thanks to research. These advances have made it possible to improve the quality of care, speed up interventions and offer more effective solutions to patients. Here is an overview of the most significant advances in emergency research:

- **Improved triage tools**: More sophisticated, evidence-based algorithms have been developed to rapidly assess the severity of patients on arrival, enabling faster, more appropriate care.
- **New biomarkers**: The discovery of new biomarkers, such as those that can detect a heart attack more quickly, has revolutionised the way in which certain cases are assessed and treated.
- **Telemedicine**: Telemedicine technologies have taken on a leading role, particularly in remote diagnosis and consultation, making care more accessible, especially in remote areas.
- **Medical simulation**: The use of high-fidelity simulation mannequins enables emergency healthcare professionals to train to manage complex situations, increasing their skills and confidence in real-life situations.
- **Point-of-care ultrasonography**: Portable ultrasound has become an essential tool for emergency physicians, enabling rapid diagnosis in situations where every second counts.
- **More effective treatments for stroke**: Thanks to research, improved protocols for the rapid management of stroke have been introduced, reducing brain damage and improving outcomes for patients.

- **Strategies to reduce overcrowding**: New methods of managing overcrowding in emergency departments have been developed, improving patient flow and reducing waiting times.
- **Pain management**: New approaches to managing acute and chronic pain, with a particular focus on opioid reduction, have been put forward thanks to research in emergency departments.
- **Psychiatric crisis intervention**: Improved assessment and intervention methods for patients in psychiatric crisis have been developed, ensuring safer and more humane care.
- **Management of cardiac arrest**: Research has also helped to optimise resuscitation techniques and protocols, improving the chances of survival and long-term results.

Research into emergency medicine has been the driving force behind many advances that have shaped modern practice, making care more efficient, rapid and patient-centred. Thanks to these advances, healthcare professionals are better equipped to meet the unique challenges of the fast-paced world of emergency medicine, and patients benefit from better quality care. Continued research is therefore essential if we are to continue to improve and innovate in this crucial area of medicine.

Chapter 12:
PREVENTION AND EDUCATION

The role of the nurse in prevention

Nurses are much more than just medical care providers. Their role also extends to prevention, a key element of public health. Prevention is one of the pillars of modern medicine, as it aims not only to treat illness, but above all to prevent it from developing in the first place. Here's how nurses play a central role in this area:

- **Education and awareness**: Nurses are often the patient's first point of contact when it comes to health issues. As such, they inform patients about the best practices to adopt to prevent illness: a balanced diet, regular physical activity, stopping smoking, etc.
- **Vaccination**: Nurses play a key role in vaccination, not only by administering vaccines, but also by raising awareness of their importance and responding to patients' concerns.
- **Early detection**: Thanks to their clinical skills, nurses can identify the first signs of certain pathologies. They then refer patients for more in-depth examinations if necessary.
- **Sexual health advice**: Nurses can also play an essential role in the prevention of sexually transmitted diseases, by advising on safe sex practices and offering screening tests.
- **Preventing nosocomial infections**: In healthcare establishments, nurses are on the front line when it comes to implementing hygiene protocols to prevent the spread of infections.
- **Monitoring chronic illnesses**: For patients suffering from chronic illnesses such as diabetes or

hypertension, the nurse provides regular monitoring, advising on diet and physical activity, and ensuring they take the right medication.

- **Mental health awareness**: Nurses are often one of the first healthcare professionals to recognise the signs of a mental health problem. They can then direct the patient to the appropriate resources and offer initial support.
- **Preventing accidents in the home**: Nurses, particularly in paediatrics and geriatrics, give advice on preventing accidents in the home, such as falls.
- **Therapeutic education**: Nurses help patients to understand their illness, the treatment prescribed and its importance, thereby improving adherence to treatment and preventing complications.
- **Promoting a healthy environment**: By understanding the social determinants of health, nurses can advise patients on how to interact positively with their environment, whether through nutrition, exercise or mental well-being.

Nurses play a key role in prevention. Through their direct contact with patients, their training and their dedication, they play a central role in promoting healthy living, preventing disease and raising awareness of healthy habits. In an era when chronic diseases are on the rise and prevention is more crucial than ever, the role of the nurse is more relevant and necessary than ever.

Educating the public
on common hazards

Public health is largely based on prevention. To ensure everyone's safety, educating the public about common hazards is crucial. Collective awareness can significantly reduce the risk of accidents and illness. Here is one approach to raising public awareness of certain common hazards:

- Smoking and alcoholism :
  - **Communicate the consequences**: highlight the dangers of smoking and alcoholism, such as heart disease, cancer and liver disease.
  - **Offer alternatives**: Offer smoking cessation programmes or group activities for those trying to reduce their alcohol consumption.
- Road safety :
  - **Responsible driving**: Raise awareness of the need to wear seatbelts, the ban on using a mobile phone at the wheel, and the dangers of driving under the influence of alcohol or drugs.
  - **Prevention for pedestrians**: Provide advice on pedestrian crossings, the importance of night-time visibility and high-risk areas.
- Falls prevention :
  - **At home**: Focus on making carpets safe, providing adequate lighting, and using aids such as grab rails.
  - **Outdoors**: Educate people about the importance of wearing appropriate footwear, especially in winter.
- Healthy eating :
  - **Avoid food poisoning**: Offer workshops on food storage and cooking.
  - **Promote a balanced diet**: Encourage the consumption of fruit and vegetables and the reduction of processed foods.
- Water safety :
  - **Learn to swim**: Offer swimming lessons for all ages.
  - **Safety equipment**: Promote the use of lifejackets and caution near deep or flowing water.

- Sun exposure :
  - **Sun protection**: Educate people about the use of sun creams, the need to wear protective hats and clothing, and the hours of exposure to be avoided.
  - **Dangers of UV**: Raise awareness of the risk of skin cancer and cataracts.
- Use of medicines :
  - **Adhering to prescriptions**: Inform people about the importance of following medical recommendations and not sharing medicines.
  - **Safe storage**: Raise awareness of the importance of keeping medicines out of the reach of children.
- Infection prevention :
  - **Hand hygiene**: Educate people about the importance of regular hand washing.
  - **Vaccination**: Raise awareness of the importance of vaccines in preventing certain serious diseases.

- Digital security :
  - **Data protection**: Inform people about the dangers of online scams and the need to protect their personal information.
  - **Responsible use**: Raise awareness, especially among young people, of the dangers of cyberbullying.
- Prevention of bites and stings:
  - **Pets**: Educate people about the importance of not disturbing animals while they are eating or sleeping.
  - **Insects and parasites**: Promote the use of repellents and appropriate clothing to protect against ticks and mosquitoes.

By raising public awareness of these common hazards, we can hope to significantly reduce the number of accidents, illnesses and deaths. Education is the first step towards a safer and healthier society.

Working with communities for prevention initiatives

One of the keys to successful prevention is collaboration between health professionals and the communities themselves. Working hand in hand with communities means that prevention messages can be adapted to the reality and specific needs of each community. Here is an outline of what such collaboration might involve:

1. Understanding the community :
It is essential to know the demographics, customs, beliefs and behaviour specific to each community. Organising meetings, interviews and discussion groups can help to identify these elements.

2. Identification of community leaders :
Every community has natural or official leaders who play a key role in mobilising members. They may be religious leaders, teachers, local councillors or other influential figures.

3. Creation of local partnerships :
Working with local organisations, schools, businesses, associations and religious groups is essential for maximum impact. These partners can provide resources, volunteers and communication channels.

4. Designing adapted programmes :
Prevention programmes need to be tailored to the specific needs of the community. If a community is particularly

affected by diabetes, for example, a prevention programme could focus on nutrition and physical activity.

5. Organisation of workshops and training courses :
These sessions can cover a variety of subjects, from CPR (cardiopulmonary resuscitation) to road safety and the prevention of infectious diseases.

6. Awareness campaigns :
Use all available means of communication, from brochures to social media, to disseminate relevant information. Involving young people in the creation of content, such as videos or posters, can be particularly effective.

7. Evaluation and feedback :
Once initiatives have been implemented, it is crucial to measure their effectiveness. This can be done through surveys, interviews or observations. Feedback from community members is essential for adjusting and improving programmes.

8. Celebrating success :
Recognising and celebrating progress strengthens community cohesion and encourages continued effort. This can be done through ceremonies, awards or community days.

9. Ensuring sustainability :
For an initiative to be sustainable, it is important to involve the community in its management and funding. This strengthens the sense of ownership and ensures that the programme will continue even without external intervention.

Ultimately, working with communities on prevention initiatives is not just about disseminating information. It's about creating solid partnerships, listening and responding to the specific needs of each community. It's a long-term investment that, when done well, can lead to significant improvements in health and well-being.

Chapter 13:
PHYSICAL WELL-BEING
AND ERGONOMICS AT WORK

Physical risks from work to emergency

The emergency department is a particularly demanding environment for the body and mind. The nurses and medical staff who work there are confronted with a variety of physical risks arising from the very nature of their work. Let's take a closer look at the aspects inherent in this particular professional setting.

1. Exposure to infectious diseases: Emergency departments see patients with a variety of conditions, including transmissible infections, on a daily basis. Workers may be exposed to viruses such as HIV, hepatitis B and C, tuberculosis, influenza and, more recently, viruses such as COVID-19.

2. Musculoskeletal injuries: Repetitive movements, such as lifting or moving patients, can lead to strain and injury. Nurses may suffer from back pain, tendonitis or other ailments linked to regular handling of patients or equipment.

3. Cuts and needlesticks: Sharp instruments, needles and other medical equipment present a risk of injury. An accidental puncture can lead to the transmission of infectious diseases.

4. Chemical hazards: Medicines, disinfectants and other chemicals used in the emergency department can be toxic if they come into direct contact with the patient or are inhaled.

5. Radiation exposure: Although radiological examinations are routinely carried out in other parts of the hospital, emergency staff may be accidentally exposed, especially if they are present during emergency procedures requiring X-rays.

6. Physical aggression: Unfortunately, emergency departments can sometimes be the scene of violence. Patients under the influence of drugs or alcohol, or those who are extremely stressed or anxious, can become aggressive.

7. Physical fatigue: Long working hours, night shifts and the relentless pace of work can lead to extreme physical fatigue, increasing the risk of medical errors and personal injury.

8. Environmental risks : Wet or contaminated floors, electrical cables and cluttered spaces can all present risks of falls or accidents for staff.

Each of the risks listed above requires specific preventive measures, whether through training, personal protective equipment, intervention protocols or ongoing awareness-raising. It is imperative that hospitals and emergency services recognise these risks and do everything possible to protect their staff, as their safety is intrinsically linked to the quality of the care they provide.

Ergonomic advice for nursing care

Ergonomics, the study of the efficiency and safety of the working environment, is of paramount importance in nursing. Faced with physically demanding tasks, the need for repetitive movements and the pressure of time, ergonomics becomes crucial to prevent injuries and ensure optimal comfort during work. Here are some ergonomic tips for nursing:

1. Use good body mechanics :
   • When lifting or moving a patient, keep your back straight, bend your knees and use the strength of your legs rather than your back.
   • Avoid bending or stretching unnecessarily; instead, get closer to what you need.

2. Suitable equipment :
   • Use lifting aids, such as slings or adjustable beds, to help move patients.
   • Make sure that chairs and workstations are at the right height to avoid awkward postures.

3. Break and stretching :
   • Take regular short breaks to stretch and move around, especially if you stay in the same position for a long time.
   • Regular stretching of the arms, legs, neck and back can help prevent tension.

4. Adapting to the environment :
   • Remove obstacles from the ground to reduce the risk of tripping.
   • Regularly place heavy or frequently used objects at a height between the hip and the chest to avoid stooping or stretching.

5. Suitable footwear :
   • Wear comfortable, well-fitting shoes with good support to reduce fatigue and the risk of falling.

6. Training and awareness :
- Take part in ergonomics training courses designed specifically for nursing.
- Keep up to date with the latest research and recommendations on ergonomics in the medical sector.

7. Ergonomic equipment :
- Use trolleys, tables and other equipment designed to reduce physical strain.
- Think about ergonomic keyboards or mice if you spend a lot of time in front of a computer.

8. Adjusting the pace of work :
- Where possible, alternate heavy tasks with lighter ones to allow your body to recover.
- Be aware of your own limits; don't be afraid to ask for help when you need it.

9. Sharing experience :
- Discuss ergonomic challenges and solutions with your colleagues to share knowledge.
- Share the tips that work for you and learn from the experience of others.

Ergonomics is not just a question of comfort, but a real necessity to ensure the safety and well-being of nurses. By following this advice and listening to their bodies, nurses can reduce their risk of injury and enjoy a longer, more satisfying career.

Maintaining good physical health long term

Physical health is the cornerstone of a balanced life lived to the full. Maintaining it is essential to our ability to enjoy life, fulfil our obligations and overcome challenges. The key lies in a proactive, ongoing and integrated approach. Here are a few tips for ensuring good physical health over the long term:

1. Eat a balanced diet:
   - Eat a diet rich in fruit, vegetables, whole grains, lean proteins and sources of healthy fats.
   - Avoid over-consumption of sugars, saturated fats and salt.

2. Exercise regularly:
   - Find an activity you enjoy, whether it's walking, swimming, dancing, yoga or any other sport.
   - Aim for at least 150 minutes of moderate activity a week.

3. Preserve your sleep :
   - Try to get 7 to 9 hours of sleep a night.
   - Adopt a regular routine for getting up and going to bed, even at weekends.

4. Manage stress :
   - Identify the sources of stress in your life and look for ways to reduce or eliminate them.
   - Practice meditation, deep breathing or other relaxation techniques.

5. Avoid risky behaviour:
   - Avoid alcohol abuse, smoking and drugs.
   - Drive carefully and always wear your seatbelt.

6. Have regular check-ups:
   - Consult your doctor regularly for check-ups and preventive tests.
   - Don't ignore unusual signs or symptoms.

7. Take care of your mental health:
   - Mental health has a strong influence on physical health. Talk about your feelings and don't hesitate to seek professional help if necessary.

8. Stay hydrated:
   - Drink at least 2 litres of water a day, more if you're active or it's hot.

9. Limit exposure to toxins :
   - Reduce the use of chemicals in your home.
   - Avoid breathing air pollutants, whether passive smoking or industrial pollution.

10. Maintain your social life :
   - A fulfilling social life is linked to better physical health. Surround yourself with positive people and stay active in your community.

By adopting these healthy habits, you create a solid framework for a long life full of vitality and well-being. Remember that maintaining good health is easier than recovering from illness or injury. Your body is your most precious possession; treat it with the respect and care it deserves.

Chapter 14:
LEGAL ASPECTS
AND RESPONSIBILITIES

Understanding legal liability as a nurse

The role of a nurse involves not only medical expertise and compassion for the well-being of patients, but also a thorough knowledge of their legal responsibilities. These responsibilities guarantee patient safety, the quality of the care provided and the protection of the rights of all those involved. Here is an overview of the main aspects of nurses' legal responsibilities.

1. Duty of care :
   * As a nurse, you have a professional duty to provide competent and appropriate care to patients. This involves following medical protocols, clinical guidelines and the ethical standards of the profession.

2. Informed consent :
   * Patients have the right to know and understand the treatments proposed to them, as well as the potential associated risks. Nurses must ensure that patients have given their informed consent prior to any medical procedure.

3. Confidentiality :
   * Nurses are obliged to protect the confidentiality of their patients' medical information. Disclosing information without appropriate consent, except in exceptional circumstances prescribed by law, may result in legal consequences.

4. Neglect :
   - If a nurse fails in their duty of care, causing harm to the patient, they can be held liable for negligence. This can have serious consequences, both professionally and legally.

5. Administration of medicines :
   - Incorrect administration of medication or failure to monitor side effects may result in legal consequences. Nurses must strictly follow medical guidelines and established protocols.

6. Precise documentation :
   - Medical records play an essential role in the delivery of care. Incorrect or incomplete documentation can not only affect the quality of care, but can also lead to legal liability.

7. Knowledge of laws and regulations :
   - Nurses must be aware of the local, regional and national laws and regulations that govern their profession. This includes knowledge of guidelines on patient rights, end-of-life care, abuse, etc.

8. Defending patients' rights :
   - Nurses have a duty to defend and protect their patients' rights, particularly in terms of dignity, autonomy and confidentiality.

9. Reporting incidents :
   - If an incident or irregularity occurs, the nurse is often required, depending on the jurisdiction, to report it to management or the relevant authorities.

10. Maintaining competence :
   - The law generally requires nurses to continue their training throughout their career to ensure that their skills and knowledge are up to date.

Understanding and respecting these legal responsibilities is essential not only for the safety and well-being of patients, but also for the protection of nurses themselves. In an ever-changing medical world, it is imperative to keep abreast of legislative and ethical changes in order to provide the best possible care.

Medical documentation: importance and good practice

Medical documentation is at the heart of the care process. It provides a clear picture of the patient's medical history, helping to ensure continuity and quality of care. Careful, complete and accurate documentation is essential not only to protect patients, but also to shield healthcare professionals from potential legal liabilities. Let's take a look at the importance of medical documentation and the best practices to adopt.

The importance of medical documentation :
- **Continuity of care**: Medical documentation enables all healthcare professionals to quickly and accurately understand a patient's medical history, current treatments and any allergies or contraindications.
- **Communication**: It facilitates communication between the various medical professionals involved, such as doctors, nurses, pharmacists and other specialists.
- **Clinical decisions**: Having access to complete medical records helps healthcare professionals to make informed decisions and avoid potential errors.
- **Legal protection**: In the event of a dispute, medical documentation serves as objective proof of patient care.

- **Research and training**: Medical records are essential resources for clinical research, enabling us to constantly improve the care we provide.

Good practice in medical documentation :
- **Accuracy**: Make sure you enter all the information accurately, without leaving out any important details.
- **Completeness**: Do not leave any fields blank. If any information is unknown or not applicable, make a clear note of this.
- **Legibility**: Whether handwritten or digital, make sure the documentation is legible. Poorly read information can lead to medical errors.
- **Objectivity**: Record only the facts and avoid subjective judgements or interpretations.
- **Updates**: Make sure that your medical records are regularly updated, particularly in the event of changes in treatment, changes in symptoms or test results.
- **Confidentiality**: Medical records contain sensitive information. Make sure they are stored securely and that only authorised people have access to them.
- **Sign and date**: Every entry in the medical record must be signed and dated, to ensure that the information can be traced.
- **Use appropriate medical terminology**: This ensures that the information is accurate and clear.
- **Correcting mistakes**: If a mistake is made, never erase or use a corrector. Draw a single line through the error, write the correction next to it and sign and date the change.
- **Retention**: Keep medical records for as long as required by local laws and regulations.

Medical documentation is much more than a simple administrative formality. It is central to medical care, ensuring patient safety and well-being while guaranteeing the quality of care. Adopting and maintaining good documentation practices is therefore a crucial responsibility for all healthcare professionals.

Managing complaints and disputes

In the midst of the hustle and bustle and complexity of emergency services, nurses are often confronted with disgruntled patients, families or even colleagues. These complaints and disputes can arise from a range of situations, from simple misunderstandings to medical errors. Handling these incidents well is essential, not only to maintain a calm working atmosphere, but also to ensure patient trust and safety.

Causes of complaints and disputes :

- **Unmet expectations**: Patients and their families may have expectations about waiting times, the care provided or the results of treatment.
- **Insufficient or inadequate communication**: A poorly informed patient may feel dissatisfied or even anxious.
- **Medical errors**: Although rare, errors can have serious physical and psychological consequences.
- **Unforeseen complications**: Even with proper care, complications can arise, leading to frustration and dissatisfaction.

Managing complaints effectively :

- **Active listening**: Take the time to listen to the complainant without interrupting. Let them express their concerns or anger. Often, being heard can ease the tension.
- **Empathy**: Show understanding and empathy for the concerns of the patient or their family. A simple "I understand why you're upset" can make a big difference.

- **Don't get defensive**: Even if you disagree, avoid getting defensive. This can make the situation worse.
- **Clarify**: Ask for details so that you understand the nature of the problem. Ask open-ended questions.
- **Provide an answer**: Give clear, honest and factual explanations. If a mistake has been made, admit it and apologise.
- **Solve**: If possible, propose solutions or corrective measures to address the concerns.
- **Document**: Make a note of all the details of the complaint and the response provided. This can be crucial in the event of escalation or subsequent litigation.

Management of formal disputes :
- **Consult your line manager**: Always inform your line manager of the situation and follow internal procedures.
- **Detailed documentation**: Make sure that all aspects of the care and complaint are carefully documented. This can be used as evidence if necessary.
- **Work with the legal department**: If the situation degenerates into litigation, work closely with your establishment's legal department to ensure that you are properly protected and advised.
- **Mediation**: In some cases, mediation can be useful in resolving disputes amicably.

To prevent complaints and disputes:
- **Improve communication**: Good communication with patients and their families can prevent many misunderstandings.
- **Ongoing training**: Regular training in interpersonal skills, medical ethics and clinical protocols can reduce errors and misunderstandings.

Never forget that every complaint or dispute is a learning opportunity. They can reveal areas for improvement, leading to better care for all patients in the future.

Chapter 15:
CONTINUING TRAINING
AND CAREER DEVELOPMENT

Training throughout your career

• Specialised training

Emergency medicine is a vast and complex field, requiring specific expertise and preparation. As front-line professionals, nurses are often exposed to a variety of cases, from the least complex to the most critical. That's why a wide range of specialised training courses are available to enhance their knowledge and skills.

1. Advanced emergency care training :
   - **ALS (Advanced Life Support):** This essential training focuses on advanced cardiopulmonary resuscitation, giving nurses the tools they need to manage life-threatening emergencies.
   - **ATLS (Advanced Trauma Life Support):** Focused on the management of the trauma patient, it offers a systematic methodology for assessing and treating injuries.
2. Paediatric training :
   - **PALS (Pediatric Advanced Life Support):** This course focuses on the management of life-threatening emergencies in children and infants.
   - **ENPC (Emergency Nursing Pediatric Course):** A programme designed for nurses to hone their skills in assessing and treating children in emergency situations.
3. Specialist maternity skills :
   - **NRP (Neonatal Resuscitation Programme):** Targeting neonatal resuscitation, this training is

essential for nurses working in emergency units with a high obstetric presence.

4. Management of psychiatric emergencies :
   - **CPI (Crisis Prevention Institute)**: It prepares nurses to interact effectively with patients in psychiatric crisis, offering de-escalation techniques.

5. Specialisation in cardiology :
   - **ACLS (Advanced Cardiac Life Support)**: This advanced training focuses on cardiac resuscitation, treatment of cardiac arrest and other cardiovascular emergencies.

6. Toxicology training :
   - Specific courses can train nurses to identify and treat overdoses, poisonings and other toxic emergencies.

7. Training in advanced emergency techniques :
   - These include skills such as the placement of central venous lines, emergency intubation and the use of specific equipment.

8. Management and leadership training :
   - For those looking to move up the ladder, training in team management, leadership or crisis management can be beneficial.

9. Further training and practical workshops :
   - Medical innovations and technological advances mean that knowledge needs to be updated on a regular basis. Practical workshops and simulations are excellent ways of improving and updating skills.

For nurses, taking one or more of these specialist courses not only means broadening their range of skills, but also improving the quality of patient care. In the hectic pace of emergency care, these skills can mean the difference between life and death, and ensure that patients in distress receive the best possible care.

• Additional qualifications and diplomas

The fast-paced and unpredictable world of medical emergencies requires nurses not only to have a solid foundation of clinical skills, but also to constantly strive to expand and update their knowledge. Fortunately, there are many additional certifications and degrees that allow nurses to further specialise and stand out in their profession.

1. Certification in emergency nursing (CEN) :
Designed specifically for emergency nurses, this certification recognises excellence in patient care in emergency situations. It covers areas such as cardiology, traumatology, paediatrics and many more.

2. Certification as a Practitioner in Intensive Care (CCRN) :
Although primarily intended for intensive care nurses, this certification is also valuable for those working in emergency departments, as it deals with the care of seriously ill or unstable patients.

3. Certification in flight nursing (CFRN) :
For nurses taking part in medical evacuation missions by helicopter or plane, this certification covers all aspects of air transport of patients.

4. Certification in Paediatric Emergency Nursing (CPEN) :
It focuses specifically on the management of paediatric patients in an emergency setting, an essential skill given the anatomical and physiological differences between adults and children.

5. University diploma in pain management :
With pain being one of the most common complaints in emergency departments, this specialised training enables nurses to acquire advanced skills in the assessment and management of pain.

6. Diploma in wound care and ostomy :
For nurses wishing to specialise in the management of wounds, ostomies and continence.

7. Certification in case management :
It prepares nurses to coordinate patient care in a holistic way, taking into account not only medical needs, but also psychosocial, financial and community needs.

8. University diploma in emergency psychiatry :
The management of patients in psychiatric crisis is a crucial aspect of emergency care, and this training course provides specialist tools for effective intervention.

9. Certifications in clinical research :
For nurses interested in the field of research, these certifications provide training in research methodologies, ethics and other aspects of conducting clinical studies.

10. Leadership and management training :
Programmes that prepare nurses for leadership roles, whether as supervisors, managers or educators.
By investing in these additional certifications and diplomas, nurses not only enhance their own skills, but also contribute to raising standards of care within the emergency department. These qualifications demonstrate a commitment to professional excellence and guarantee optimum care for patients in emergency situations.

Career prospects

• Becoming a head nurse
Becoming head nurse in the emergency department is a natural progression for many experienced nurses, marking the transition from direct care delivery to a position of leadership and management. The Chief Nurse plays a vital

role in coordinating care, managing resources and providing strategic direction to the Emergency Department. It's a demanding role, but also an incredibly rewarding one.

The path to leadership :
The journey to the role of Chief Nurse usually begins in the field. Years spent providing direct patient care forge an intimate understanding of the department's challenges and needs. This experience is essential for making informed decisions as a leader.

Skills and qualities required:
In addition to clinical skills, a nurse leader must have management, communication and leadership skills. The ability to manage teams, resolve conflicts, plan strategically and ensure fluid communication is crucial.

Responsibilities:
A head nurse generally supervises all the nursing staff in the department, manages schedules, coordinates ongoing training, acts as a liaison between the nursing staff and hospital management, and plays an active role in strategic and budgetary decisions.

Training and education :
While clinical experience is fundamental, additional training in management or administration is often recommended. Many nurse leaders pursue masters degrees in nursing administration or health management to hone their leadership skills.

Challenges and rewards :
While the role of head nurse can be stressful, with the pressure of decision-making and responsibility for an entire department, it is also extremely rewarding. Fostering a positive culture, promoting excellence in care, and seeing your team flourish are all rewarding aspects of the job.

The future of the role :
With the constant evolution of the medical world, the role of the head nurse is destined to evolve. Technology, medical innovations and changes in healthcare management will require continuous adaptation and training.

Becoming a chief nurse is an ambitious goal, but for those who are up for the challenge, it's an opportunity to make a real difference to the quality of care delivered in emergency departments and to the lives of their nursing colleagues.

• Possible specialisations

The world of nursing is vast, and emergency medicine is just one of the many specialties a nurse can specialise in. While the emergency department offers solid, versatile training, there are other areas where nurses can hone their skills and develop particular expertise. Here's an overview of possible specialisations after experience in the emergency department:

1. Intensive care :
Nurses specialising in intensive care look after seriously ill or unstable patients who require constant monitoring. This role requires a deep understanding of human physiology and a command of advanced medical equipment.

2. Cardiology :
Nurses specialising in cardiology care for patients suffering from heart disease. They may work in coronary care units, catheterisation laboratories or specialist clinics.

3. Paediatrics :
Paediatric nurses specialise in caring for children from birth to adolescence. They must understand the specificities of the development and growth of this population.

4. Obstetrics and gynaecology :
Here, nurses focus on women's reproductive health, pregnancy, childbirth and post-partum care.

5. Psychiatry :
In this field, nurses work with patients suffering from mental disorders or addiction, in hospital or on an outpatient basis.

6. Oncology :
Oncology nurses specialise in the care of cancer patients, including the administration of chemotherapy and symptom management.

7. Traumatology :
This speciality focuses on the care of patients who have suffered major trauma, whether accidental or intentional.

8. Geriatrics :
Geriatric nurses focus on caring for the elderly, taking into account the unique aspects of ageing.

9. Clinical research :
Research nurses design and implement clinical studies to test new medical interventions.

10. Education :
Nurse educators teach future health professionals, whether in nursing schools, hospitals or universities.

11. Management :
Some nurses choose to move into management positions, supervising teams, units or even entire establishments.

12. Community health :
These nurses work outside hospitals, in community clinics, schools or homes, focusing on prevention and education.

Each specialisation has its own challenges and rewards, but all enable nurses to make a significant contribution to the health and well-being of patients. It is often advisable to pursue specific training and certification for each of these specialties to ensure competent and up-to-date practice.

Chapter 16:
SOME EXAMPLES OF TESTIMONIALS
AND ANECDOTES FROM THE FIELD

Unforgettable days:
Tales of extreme situations

Life in an emergency department is unpredictable. Every day brings its share of challenges, emotions and moments that leave a lasting impression on nurses. Here are a few stories that illustrate the range of extreme situations that nurses can face:

The night of the bus crash:
It was a typical evening when the emergency bell rang. A bus full of students returning from a school trip had been involved in a serious accident on the motorway. Ambulances were pouring in, carrying teenagers in a state of shock, seriously injured teachers and passengers from other vehicles involved. The emergency team mobilised as a close-knit unit, triaging and treating patients, calling on internal and external resources, while managing the anguish of families and friends arriving in search of news. It was a stark reminder of the fragility of life and the importance of a close-knit, efficient team.

Flash flooding :
When a flash flood hit the area, the hospital became a refuge for many displaced people. The emergency department was overwhelmed, not only by flood-related injuries, but also by patients with chronic conditions whose treatment had been interrupted by the disaster. Nurses adapted, transforming non-medical areas into care zones,

distributing medicines, clothing and food, and offering emotional support to those who had lost everything.

A baby's heart attack :
One morning, a mother arrived in panic with her six-month-old baby in her arms, blue and unresponsive. The nurses immediately began cardiopulmonary resuscitation. While some members of the team worked desperately to stabilise the little patient, others supported the collapsed mother. Thanks to their rapid intervention, the baby was resuscitated and transferred to paediatric intensive care. That day, every second counted.

Stabbing:
In mid-afternoon, a man arrived, bloodied, the victim of a stabbing during an altercation. As the nurses worked to stabilise his injuries, they also had to manage the palpable tension, as the assailant, who had also been injured, had been brought to the same emergency room. Staff had to maintain safety while providing quality care to all patients.

These stories illustrate the variety and intensity of situations with which emergency nurses can be confronted. Each situation requires not only clinical skills, but also the ability to manage stress, work as part of a team and show compassion. These unforgettable days build character, remind us of the importance of the profession and leave indelible memories.

Small victories:
Moments of joy and gratitude

In the hustle and bustle of the emergency department, every day is a whirlwind of emotions. Amongst the most difficult moments, there are also bursts of joy, moments of gratitude that warm the heart and remind us why so many nurses choose this profession despite its challenges. These small victories are the rays of sunshine that pierce the darkness of the darkest days.

A child's glimmer of hope :
A seven-year-old boy had been in a bicycle accident and suffered multiple fractures. Every day, despite his pain, he tried to smile and laugh with the care team. The moment when, after weeks of rehabilitation, he took his first hesitant steps in the corridor with the help of the nurses, remains engraved as a triumph on the faces of all those present.

Silent recognition :
An elderly man with a stroke had difficulty communicating. Every interaction was an ordeal for him. One day, after one of the nurses had taken the time to shave and wash him, he put his hand on hers, squeezing it gently, his eyes shining with a gratitude he couldn't express in words.

The return of a cured patient:
A young woman, admitted for serious drug poisoning in a desperate act, had spent days in intensive care. The nurses took turns at her bedside, supporting her in her most vulnerable moments. Months later, she returned, beaming, to thank the team, telling them that it was their compassion and support that had helped her regain the will to live.
Surprise birthday party :

Knowing that a little girl who had been in hospital for a long time was going to spend her birthday in hospital, the emergency team got together to organise a surprise party for her. Seeing her blow out her candles, surrounded by nurses singing to her, was a reminder that recovery is measured not just in medicines and treatments, but also in shared moments of joy.

These moments of happiness and recognition, although sometimes brief, have a lasting impact. They remind nurses of the profound humanity of their work, the beauty of the bonds they forge with their patients, and the priceless value of small victories in the midst of chaos. In these moments, the emergency department becomes a place not only of physical healing, but also of hope and human connection.

Chapter 17:
CONCLUSION: THE NURSE, EMERGENCY PILLAR

Essential qualities the emergency nurse

Emergency nurses are confronted on a daily basis with unexpected and sometimes critical situations, and find themselves at the crossroads between the patient's immediate needs and medical requirements. This position requires a unique combination of technical, emotional and interpersonal qualities. In this demanding profession, certain qualities stand out as being of crucial importance.

Adaptability:
In an emergency, no two days are alike. Nurses must constantly adapt to changing situations, whether it's new admissions, unexpected medical cases or major crises. This ability to evolve and reposition quickly is essential if they are to respond effectively to patients' needs.

Emotional resilience:
In the face of suffering, distress and even death, emergency nurses must be emotionally robust. They must be able to manage their own emotions while offering support and compassion to patients and their families.

Rapid decision-making:
In a context where every second counts, emergency nurses must be able to make decisions quickly, based on their clinical judgement, training and experience.

Communication:
Knowing how to communicate clearly with doctors, other

nurses, and above all with patients and their families, is essential. This communication must be both precise from a medical point of view and reassuring from a human point of view.

Team spirit:
The emergency department is an environment where collaboration is essential. Emergency nurses must be able to work in harmony with a multidisciplinary team, sharing information and responsibilities for the well-being of the patient.

The ability to learn continuously:
Medicine is constantly evolving. To keep abreast of the latest techniques and recommendations, nurses need to be eager to learn, ready to train and adapt to new methods and technologies.

Organisation:
In the whirlwind of emergencies, the ability to prioritise, manage time and coordinate several tasks simultaneously is crucial.

Empathy:
Although the technical aspect is essential, the human dimension remains at the heart of the profession. Understanding and connecting with patients, feeling and responding to their emotional needs, is an essential quality for an emergency nurse.

Integrity:
In an environment where trust is vital, nurses must demonstrate impeccable ethics, guaranteeing patient safety and respect.

Patience:
Even in an emergency, there will be moments of waiting,

moments when the nurse will have to explain, reassure or simply be present. Patience is therefore an invaluable asset.

Each of these qualities, cultivated and refined over time, makes the emergency nurse an indispensable professional, a pillar on which the rapid and effective care of patients in distress rests.

Looking to the future:
The emergencies of tomorrow

The world of healthcare is constantly changing, driven by technological advances, scientific discoveries and social transformations. And emergency departments, the crucial entry point to the healthcare system, are no exception. So what might the emergency department of tomorrow look like? Let's take a closer look.

The integration of telemedicine:
While telemedicine is gaining ground in many medical fields, it is set to play a growing role in emergency departments. Remote consultations could make it possible to quickly assess the seriousness of a situation, direct patients to the right service or relieve waiting room congestion.

Cutting-edge technologies:
Artificial intelligence and algorithms could help prioritise patients according to the seriousness of their condition. Virtual reality tools could be used for ongoing team training or to simulate complex emergency scenarios. Robotics could also play a role, for example in dispensing medicines or assisting with certain procedures.

A patient-centred environment:
Taking into account patients' well-being will not be limited solely to their physical state of health. More comfortable spaces, better communication, interactive tools to inform patients and their families, and a holistic approach to care are all elements that could become widespread.

The importance of sustainable development:
Taking into account the environmental impact of emergency services will be crucial. This could mean optimising resources, using environmentally-friendly materials or installing renewable energy systems.

Strengthened multidisciplinary teams:
Collaboration between healthcare professionals will be further developed, for example by integrating mental health specialists directly into emergency departments, or by strengthening the link between general practitioners and emergency departments.

Appropriate continuing training:
Faced with an ever-changing medical world, the training of emergency nurses and doctors will be dynamic, using the latest technologies and adapting rapidly to new health issues.

Specialist emergency departments:
In addition to the paediatric and cardiology emergency departments that already exist, we could see the emergence of emergency departments dedicated to specific pathologies, offering ultra-specialised care.

Optimised information systems:
Interconnected, secure electronic medical records will make it easier to share information, optimising the patient's care pathway and guaranteeing better continuity of care.

While the future holds great promise, it will also bring its share of challenges. Tomorrow's emergency services will have to be up to the challenge, combining medical excellence with humanity, to best meet the needs of patients in a constantly changing world.

www.ingramcontent.com/pod-product-compliance
Lightning Source LLC
Chambersburg PA
CBHW062322290526
45794CB00005B/1860